Series Title: Vitamin D and Your Body
Volume Title: Why Does Vitamin D Matter?

Edited By

J. Ruth Wu-Wong

Department of Pharmacy Practice
University of Illinois, Chicago
USA

eBooks End User License Agreement

CONTENTS

FOREWORD

Vitamin D was discovered in the 1920s as a substance in cod liver oil that cured sick dogs of a bone disorder called rickets. Because it was proven to be something different than Vitamin A which had also been characterized in cod liver oil, and a vitamin B and C had already been claimed, the new substance was called vitamin D. We have come a long way! We now recognize the pluripotency of vitamin D and as more has been learned in recent years about the biology of vitamin D it continues to fascinate scientists and spur new discovery. Thus, this eBook is a timely review of science and medical knowledge underpinning our current understanding of vitamin D and what the future might hold as we learn to apply that new knowledge.

In recent years, vitamin D has been commonly referenced in the lay press. In particular, the question of how to deal with vitamin D deficiency as a public health concern has been frequently in the news. At the same time public and medical awareness has increased of the potential health consequences vitamin D deficiency or insufficiency, depending on how one wants to define it, a growing body of data is focused on the potential pharmaceutical applications of vitamin D therapy. Certainly, this aspect has been facilitated by discovery and development of several chemical analogs of vitamin D and their dramatic utility in treatment of secondary hyperparathyroidism associated with endstage renal disease, a mineral abnormality commonly associated with kidney disease. As this eBook highlights, there is increasing clinical evidence to suggest pharmacological therapy with vitamin D analogs, or vitamin D receptor modulators (VDRMs) as we prefer to call them, may have significant benefit from beyond treatment of secondary hyperparathyroidism.

This eBook reviews the history of vitamin D, current medical practice, and recent advances in our understanding of vitamin D's important role beyond mineral metabolism. In particular, its importance to cardiovascular health is made clear. This relationship is most evident in patients who suffer from chronic kidney disease (CKD). The progressive and irreversible nature of CKD is strongly associated with increased risk of cardiovascular disease and mortality. Unfortunately, the global prevalence of CKD is rapidly growing due to the epidemic of type 2 diabetes, and an aging population. The associated costs of treating these patients, especially in the later stages of disease, represent a large and growing health care burden that cannot be sustained, demanding new treatment and perhaps more aggressive treatment with existing therapeutic approaches.

Each of the authors are experts actively engaged in vitamin D research. Their chapters highlight the continuing advances being made in discovery and development of novel VDRM drugs which have great potential to improve the lives of many patients suffering from CKD, and other diseases of vitamin D deficiency. This volume will serve as a useful guide to both experienced and novice vitamin D researchers and clinicians, and to those generally interested and staying current with an active area of science that has broad implications on human health.

Read, learn and do!

Terry Opgenorth
CEO, Vidasym
Chicago
USA

PREFACE

Many eBooks have been published on the subject of vitamin D. Considering the important role vitamin D plays in human health, perhaps the plan to construct a series of eBooks on the subject of vitamin D is still worth pursuing, although the task is certainly daunting and at the same time exciting. This eBook is the first in the series and it aims to explore why vitamin D matters.

The first chapter offers the readers a brief history of the vitamin D field. It will become obvious to the readers that this is a pretty "ancient" field and many studies have been conducted in the field. The second chapter follows by detailing how vitamin D works, which shall also be accessible to a large class of readers with some scientific background.

Numerous epidemiological studies have been conducted to investigate the outcome of vitamin D deficiency and the effects of vitamin D supplementation. Chapter 3 contains a detailed account of the available data on epidemiology to help the readers understand more about the role of vitamin D in various disease states. After learning about the importance of vitamin D, the readers may wonder how much vitamin D is required to maintain good health and whether they shall increase their vitamin D intake. In Chapter 4, the issue of vitamin D supplementation is addressed from different angles.

It is important to note that vitamin D and its analogs are currently used to treat various diseases. Chapter 5 provides a comprehensive report on various vitamin D analogs currently on the market or in development. Chapter 6 continues by exploring the possibility of developing this class of compounds for additional indications.

Chapter 7 summarizes the topics discussed in the previous chapters and attempts to pin down the unresolved issues in the vitamin D field and also projects what to expect in the future.

We hope the readers will find this eBook informative, not only from the scientific point of view, but also from the potential applications of the knowledge into one's daily life. It is the authors' sincere wish that the eBook will arouse interest among young people to consider a career in biochemical/medical research, especially in the field of vitamin D.

We would like to thank Dr. Terry Opgenorth for writing the foreword and Bentham Science Publishers for their support and efforts.

J. Ruth Wu-Wong
University of Illinois at Chicago
Chicago
USA

List of Contributors

Masahide Mizobuchi
Department of Medicine, Division of Nephrology, Showa University School of Medicine, Tokyo, Japan. E-mail: mizobu@med.showa-u.ac.jp

Petya Valcheva and Jose M Valdivielso
Laboratorio de Investigación Hospital Universitario Arnau de Vilanova, IRBLLEIDA. Rovira Roure 80, Lleida. Spain. E-mail: valdivielso@medicina.udl.es

Csaba P. Kovesdy
Division of Nephrology, Salem Veterans Affairs Medical Center, 1970 Roanoke Blvd., Salem, Virginia 24153, USA. E-mail: csaba.kovesdy@va.gov

Alan Lau and Yee Ming Lee
College of Pharmacy, University of Illinois at Chicago, Chicago, IL, 60612, USA. E-mail: alanlau@uic.edu; ylee227@uic.edu

Gui-Dong Zhu
Cancer Research, GPRD, Abbott Laboratories, 100 Abbott Park Rd., Abbott Park , IL , 60064 , USA . E-mail: gui-dong.zhu@abbott.com

Alex Brown
Department of Medicine, Washington University School of Medicine, St. Louis, MO, 63130, USA. E-mail: ABROWN@DOM.wustl.edu

J. Ruth Wu-Wong
Department of Pharmacy Practice, College of Pharmacy, University of Illinois at Chicago, Chicago, IL. 60612, USA. E-mail: jrwuwong@uic.edu

A Brief History of the Vitamin D Field

Masahide Mizobuchi[*]

Division of Nephrology, Department of Medicine, Showa University School of Medicine, Japan

Abstract: The discovery of the vitamin D system, which plays an important role in maintaining the health of living beings, has made significant contributions to the medical field. Immediately after the discovery, it was postulated that vitamin D (cholecalciferol or ergocalciferol) was not active, and did not have any physiological function. It was subsequently found that vitamin D needs to be metabolized in the liver and kidney by hydroxylation to be transformed into an active form. Subsequently it was shown that most of the physiological functions of the active form of vitamin D are mediated by a nuclear receptor, the vitamin D receptor (VDR), to exert genomic actions to control expression of various VDR target genes. Furthermore, although the active form of vitamin D was originally considered to be mainly a hormone that regulates mineral metabolism, it is now recognized that active vitamin D is a hormone involved in modulating numerous physiological functions based on the wide distribution of VDR in various cells and tissues in the human body. This recognition is supported by many studies that demonstrate the correlation between abnormal vitamin D metabolism and numerous pathological conditions. In chronic kidney disease (CKD) patients with impaired vitamin D metabolism, the most significant cause of death is cardiovascular complications, suggesting an important role of the vitamin D-VDR axis in maintaining cardiovascular function. Thus, in addition to the development of vitamin D analogs for the treatment of bone disease and hyperparathyroidism secondary to CKD, the application of vitamin D analogs for treating cardiovascular disease in CKD has been attracting attention.

Keywords: Calcitriol, cholecalciferol, CYP24A1, CYP27B1, 7-dehydrocholesterol, ergocalciferol, vitamin D, active vitamin D, vitamin D receptor, vitamin D response element (VDRE).

INTRODUCTION

The identification of the active metabolite of vitamin D, 1,25-dihydroxyvitamin D, by Lawson *et al.* in the 1970s brought in the first golden age for vitamin D research [1, 2]. In the 1980s, the effect of active vitamin D on inducing cell differentiation was discovered, suggesting that vitamin D not only modulates mineral homeostasis, but also regulates various cell functions. In the late 1980s, the vitamin D receptor (VDR) was cloned [3], and VDR was recognized as the causal gene for vitamin D-dependent Type II rickets [4]. In addition, the development of the VDR gene-deficient mouse [5, 6] led to the discovery that activation of VDR is essential for the effects of active vitamin D. In 1997, 25-hydroxyvitamin D_3 1-alpha-hydroxylase (CYP27B1, 1α-hydroxylase), which controls the last phase of vitamin D activation, was identified [7]. The discovery of VDR and CYP27B1 brought in another new phase in the vitamin D field. At the same time, many vitamin D derivatives with different actions were synthesized. These derivatives seem to exhibit tissue-specific actions, depending on their differential binding modes to the VDR. Thereafter, a new endeavor began that focused on developing vitamin D analogs for clinical use.

THE DISCOVERY OF ACTIVE VITAMIN D

In the human body, 1 to 2 g of cholesterol is synthesized in the skin each day from its precursor, 7-dehydrocholesterol (provitamin D_3 or pro D_3). While a majority of cholesterols are synthesized in the liver, some cholesterols such as 7-dehydrocholesterol are made in the skin. When 7-dehydrocholesterol that is formed in epidermal cells in the skin is irradiated with ultraviolet light-B, a bond is specifically cleaved *via* photofragmentation between Carbon 9 and 10 in the B-ring (see Fig. **1**) to form previtamin D_3, which is

*Address correspondence to Masahide Mizobuchi: Department of Medicine, Division of Nephrology, Showa University School of Medicine, Tokyo, Japan. E-mail: mizobu@med.showa-u.ac.jp

J. Ruth Wu-Wong (Ed)

converted to vitamin D_3 (cholecalciferol) by isomerization. The structural difference between steroid hormones and vitamin D_3, both made from cholesterol, is in their side chains. While steroid hormones are synthesized through removal of the side chains, the side chain of vitamin D_3 remains intact. For more information on how vitamin D is made in the skin, please see subsequent chapters. Vitamin D synthesized from cholesterol in the human body is called vitamin D_3. Another major form of vitamin D, vitamin D_2 (ergocalciferol), is produced by invertebrates, fungi and plants in response to UV irradiation, but not found in vertebrates. The side chain of vitamin D_2 contains a double bond between Carbon 22 and 23 and a methyl group on Carbon 24 as shown in Fig. **1**. In mammals, vitamin D_2 seems to have the same bioactivity and metabolic pathway as vitamin D_3 (1 U = 0.025 µg) [8], although the subject is still being investigated (see subsequent chapters for more details). Avian species, on the other hand, can only utilize vitamin D_3. Chickens, in particular, require a large amount of vitamin D_3 for egg production.

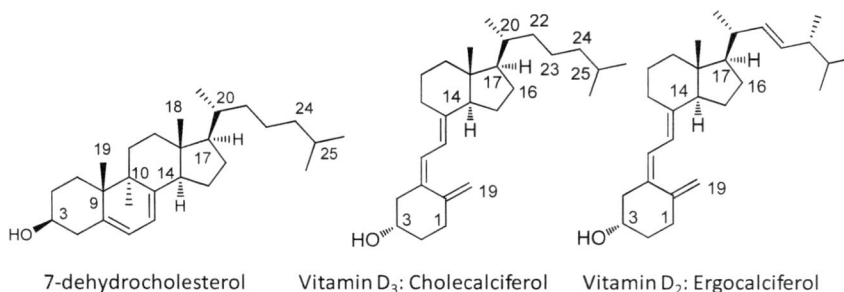

7-dehydrocholesterol   Vitamin D_3: Cholecalciferol   Vitamin D_2: Ergocalciferol

Figure 1: Structures of 7-Dehydrocholesterol, Vitamin D_3 and D_2

According to Mosby's Medical Dictionary, the definition of vitamin is as follows: "any of various organic compounds that are needed in small amounts for normal growth and activity of the body. Vitamins cannot be synthesized by the body, but are found naturally in foods obtained from plants and animals". In this regard, vitamin D is not a 'vitamin'. The possible reason why vitamin D is called a 'vitamin' is that the amount of vitamin D_3 synthesized in the skin is insufficient for the body, and additional sources are required to avoid vitamin D deficiency (hypovitaminosis D). The synthesis of vitamin D in the skin is influenced by skin color, sunshine duration, and the strength of the sun light. It has been demonstrated that people who live in areas with short sunshine duration easily develop hypovitaminosis D. Thus, it is highly recommended that additional vitamin D shall be obtained from plants and animals as a micronutrient. Very early on it was known that vitamin D was linked to bone health. Bone disorders due to vitamin D insufficiency are referred to as rickets in children and osteomalacia in adults who have an epiphyseal line.

The next important development in the vitamin D field was the discovery that vitamin D by itself is not active, but needs to be metabolized to form the active form, which increases serum calcium (Ca) levels by stimulating intestinal Ca^{2+} absorption and bone resorption [9, 10]. Evidence shows that vitamin D does not act directly on the small intestine but it is metabolized elsewhere and its active metabolite then acts on the intestine. Studies using radiochromatography showed that tissues (small intestine, liver, blood, and bone) obtained from vitamin D deficient rats injected with tritium-labeled vitamin D exhibited four peaks (Peak I to IV) of radioactivity [11]. Peak III was the unmodified vitamin D [12], while Peak I was unequivocally identified as an ester of vitamin D [13]. The Peak IV metabolite fraction was the major form found in the tissues 24 hours after dosing [11]. Peaks I and II remained as small peaks regardless of dosage or time after dosing and were presumed to be biological fragments [14]. The Peak IV fraction proved to be as active as, and probably more effective than, the parent vitamin D in increasing bone resorption and stimulating intestinal Ca^{2+} transport [11, 14]. These results suggested that the Peak IV fraction contained the active form of vitamin D. Mass spectrometry studies revealed that while vitamin D_3 had a molecular weight of 384, the molecular weight of the Peak IV metabolite was 400, indicating the presence of one additional hydroxyl functional group. Ultimately, it was called 25-hydroxyvitamin D_3 (25-hydroxycholecalciferol, 25(OH)D_3) since the OH was located at the 25 position [15]. By a similar, but somewhat different procedure, the metabolite from ergocalciferol was also isolated, and subsequently identified as 25-hydroxyergocalciferol [16]. Of great interest was the biological activity of 25(OH)D_3. Based upon the antirachitic assay, $25(OH)D_3$ is 1.5 times more active than vitamin D_3 (cholecalciferol) [17]. When $25(OH)D_3$ was tested for its ability to stimulate intestinal Ca^{2+} transport, it was not only more effective, but also produced a response faster than did a similar dose of vitamin D_3 [17]. Similar results were obtained when the bone mineralization action of vitamin D_3 was examined; the response for $25(OH)D_3$ was greater [17]. Assuming that $25(OH)D_3$ was the active form of vitamin D_3, these data suggested that ~6 hours was required to convert vitamin D_3 to $25(OH)D_3$, accounting for a major portion of the lag time in the vitamin D action. These results seemed to suggest that $25(OH)D_3$ was the metabolically active form of vitamin D_3. Further studies testing the simultaneous administration of the two radioactive substances, [4-^{14}C]cholecalciferol and [1-^{3}H]cholecalciferol, to the vitamin D-deficient chicks revealed the presence of vitamin D_3, $25(OH)D_3$, and a further metabolic product of vitamin D_3 more polar than $25(OH)D_3$ in multiple organs including blood, liver, intestine, kidney and bone [18]. This highly polar metabolite proved to be more biologically active and acted more rapidly than $25(OH)D_3$. Finally the polar metabolite was identified and termed $1\alpha,25$-dihydroxyvitamin D_3 ($1,25(OH)_2D_3$, calcitriol).

THE DISCOVERY OF THE VITAMIN D METABOLIC PATHWAY

As mentioned above, it was only after a series of studies using radiolabeled vitamin D, a clear concept finally emerged that vitamin D is not active, and needs to be metabolized *in vivo* to become active. The activation of vitamin D involving two-step hydroxylation to produce the final active hormone was first discovered in animals [19]. The first step of hydroxylation at the Carbon 25 position occurs mainly in the liver and, to a lesser degree, in several other tissues. This step takes place in both microsomes and mitchondria [20-22]. The liver mitochondrial cytochrome P450 enzyme (25-hydroxylase, CYP27A1) has the ability to hydroxylate vitamin D at high concentrations [23]. However, CYP27A1-null mice exhibit no significant changes in the serum 25(OH)D levels [24], suggesting that this enzyme, although the most well-characterized CYP27A1, may not be the only 25-hydroxylase capable of hydroxylating vitamin D at the 25th C-position. Thus, the physiological importance of this enzyme remains to be determined. The product of the 25-hydroxylation step, 25(OH)D, is the major form of vitamin D in the blood, with normal concentrations ranging from 25-35 ng/mL [25]. One of the reasons that 25(OH)D is present at a much higher concentration in circulation than $1,25(OH)_2D$ (*i.e.*, 20-60 pg/mL) is partly due to its stability, which is likely due to its strong affinity for the vitamin D-binding protein (DBP) in the blood.

The second step is 1α-hydroxylation of 25(OH)D by CYP27B1, which occurs mainly in the kidney and, to a lesser degree, in several other tissues, resulting in the active form of vitamin D, $1,25(OH)_2D$ (calcitriol). For more information on how vitamin D is converted into calcitriol, please see Chapter 5. Although purification of CYP27B1 has been attempted using proximal tubules as the source, its existence was not confirmed until 1997 [7, 26, 27]. This enzyme was classified as a member of the P450 family that exhibits activity dependent upon both adrenodoxin and adrenodoxin reductase. Although CYP27B1 plays a specific role in the synthesis of $1,25(OH)_2D$, the enzyme itself is controlled in a negative feedback mechanism by $1,25(OH)_2D$. It has been suggested that $1,25(OH)_2D$ inhibits the expression of CYP27B1 gene *via* the activation of VDR. Furthermore, the activity of CYP27B1 is modulated by the actions of PTH and calcitonin involved in bone metabolism and by a spike in blood concentrations of Ca^{2+} and phosphorus (P), all of which are involved in maintaining calcium homeostasis [28, 29]. The expression of CYP27B1 is inhibited by various factors at the transcriptional level [30-34] as shown in Table **1**.

Table 1: Regulators of CYP27B1

Positive regulator	Negative regulator
PTH	$1,25(OH)_2D_3$
Calcitonin	Ca
Sex hormone	P
Prolactin (PRL)	Thyroid hormone
Growth hormone (GH)	Glucocorticoid
Gestation	H^+
	FGF-23

PTH: parathyroid hormone, Ca: calcium, P: phosphorus, FGF: fibroblast growth factor.

CYP27B1 is mainly expressed in the kidney, but its expression has also been demonstrated in the placenta, osteoblast, macrophage, keratinocyte, vascular smooth muscle cell, *etc.* [35, 36]. The expression level of CYP27B1 in the extra-renal tissues is extremely low, and its physiological function is still under intense investigation. CYP27B1 is responsible for vitamin D dependent Type I rickets [37]. At the same time, mice lacking the CYP27B1 gene also exhibited growth impairment and other systemic disorders, in addition to rickets and osteomalacia, similar to vitamin D dependent type I rickets. In the mouse lacking the CYP27B1 gene, the blood concentration of $1,25(OH)_2D$ is not detectable, and an abnormal increase in PTH is observed. As a comparison, in VDR gene-deficient mice, the blood concentration of $1,25(OH)_2D$ increases by tenfold or more [5]. Furthermore, secondary hyperparathyroidism is improved in these CYP27B1-deficient mice when calcitriol, high calcium, high phosphorus, and/or or high lactose are administered [38].

While CYP27B1 converts $25(OH)D$ into the active metabolite $1,25(OH)_2D$, CYP24A1 (1,25-dihydroxyvitamin D_3 24-hydroxylase or 24-hydroxylase) decomposes $25(OH)D$ and $1,25(OH)_2D$ to inactivate metabolites by hydroxylating the molecules at the 24th position. The CYP24A1 gene is expressed in many different tissues including proximal tubular cells, small intestine and bone. The CYP24A1 activity is induced in the small intestine by $1,25(OH)_2D$, and the metabolism and decomposition of $1,25(OH)_2D$ in the small intestine is extremely important for the regulation of Ca^{2+} absorption. The Ca^{2+} concentration in the blood is strictly controlled between 9 and 10 mg/dL. As one of the important mechanisms for regulating Ca^{2+} homeostasis, CYP27B1 and CYP24A1 activities compete to maintain a tight range of the $1,25(OH)_2D$ concentration in blood. The CYP27B1 activity is increased when the concentrations of $1,25(OH)_2D$ and Ca^{2+} are decreased in the blood. As soon as the blood concentrations of $1,25(OH)_2D$ and Ca^{2+} are restored, the CYP24A1 activity increases, exhibiting an inverse correlation between these two enzyme activities. Both enzymes have vitamin D response element (VDRE) in their promoter region, indicating that the expression of both enzymes is controlled at the level of gene expression by VDR as shown in Fig. **2**.

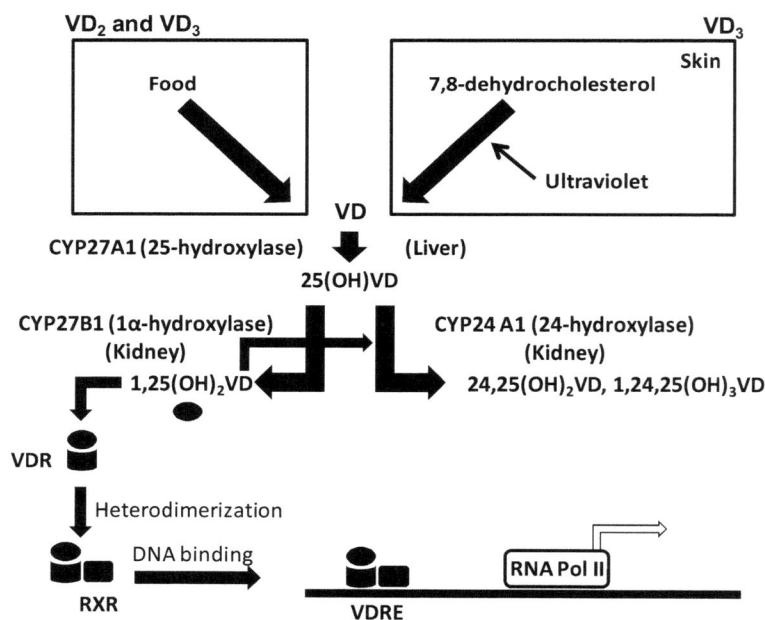

Figure 2: Vitamin D (cholecalciferol and ergocalciferol) is hydroxylated at the 25th position in the liver by CYP27A1 (25-hydroxylase) into 25-hydroxyvitamin D ($25(OH)D$), which is further hydroxylated at the 1st or 24th position in the kidney into 1,25-dihydroxyvitamin D ($1,25(OH)_2D$) or 24,25-dihydroxyvitamin D ($24,25(OH)_2D$) by CYP27B1 or CYP24A1, respectively. CYP27A1, CYP27B1, and CYP24A1 regulate the concentration of active vitamin D. $1,25(OH)_2D$ binds to its receptor, the vitamin D receptor (VDR). $1,25(OH)_2D$-activated VDR binds to its partner, the retinoic X receptor (RXR, heterodimerization), which then binds to vitamin D response element (VDRE) in the promoter region of VDR-responsive genes (DNA binding) to regulate the transcription of VDR-responsive genes by RNA polymerase II (transcriptional regulation).

In the late 1980s, the VDR was successfully cloned. The VDR is classified into the nuclear receptor superfamily. Ligand-bound VDR becomes activated and recruits cofactors such as RXR, which then binds to VDRE in the promoter of the VDR targeted genes to regulate gene expression. VDR is expressed in a wide range of tissues (Table **2**), suggesting that VDR may be involved in regulating many physiological functions.

Table 2: VDR distribution in the human body [25]

Endocrine system
Parathyroid gland, Thyroid gland, Kidney, Adrenal gland,
Pituitary gland, Breast
Cardiovascular system
Heart, Vessel
Central nerve system
Brain, Nerve
Respiratory system
Lung
Digestive system
Esophagus, Stomach, Small intestine, Colon, Liver, Pancreas
Skeletal musculature
Bone, Muscle
Urinary and productive system
Prostate, Testis, Ovary, Uterus
Lymphoreticular system
Thymus, Lymphocyte, Macrophage
Skin tissue
Skin, Hair

THE DISCOVERY OF VDR FUNCTIONS

Many data have shown that vitamin D-dependent type II rickets involve abnormal VDR function. In this disease high $1,25(OH)_2D$ levels are observed, in addition to decreased intestinal absorption of Ca^{2+} and P due to defective VDR and vitamin D resistance [4]. Furthermore, hair loss has been confirmed in approximately 67% of the families with the defective VDR gene although no such hair loss is seen in patients with other types of rickets. In 1997, the VDR gene-deficient mouse was generated [5, 6]. In the VDR-knockout mice, blood concentrations of Ca^{2+} and P are maintained normally from after birth to the weaning period at 3 weeks of age, but typical symptoms of rickets develop after the weaning period. Since no abnormalities occur during the lactation period, and Ca^{2+} supplementation rescues some of the abnormal bone phenotypes, it has been suggested that the primary role of VDR in maintaining bone metabolism might occur *via* its indirect action on promoting absorption of Ca^{2+} and P from the intestinal canal [39].

Data from several pre-clinical studies reveal additional roles for the vitamin D-VDR axis beyond regulation of mineral metabolism. The VDR-knockout mice exhibit increased blood pressure and left ventricular hypertrophy (LVH), and increased levels of renin mRNA in myocardial tissues and increased angiotension II levels in the blood. The results from the VDR-knockout mice are consistent with previous publications that there is an inverse correlation between blood concentrations of $1,25(OH)_2D$ and plasma renin activity in patients with essential hypertension [40, 41]. Recent studies further confirm that activated VDR, *via* a complex mechanism to modulate the promoter region of the renin gene, directly inhibits renin expression, thus playing a crucial role in regulating the renin-angiotensin system (RAS) to control cardiac function [42, 43]. In addition, it was also shown in a pre-clinical study that different vitamin D analogs may have different effects on renin expression [44]. Additional studies demonstrated that activated VDR not only controls RAS, but also regulates the expression of genes involved in cell-cycle regulation, and hypertrophy and apoptosis of cardiomyocytes [45]. Recently, it was shown that paricalcitol could improve oxidative stress in cardiac muscle in the 5/6 nephrectomized rats, an animal model with renal insufficiency [46]. When renal insufficiency was induced in the low-density lipoprotein receptor (LDLR) knockout mice fed a high-fat diet, atheromatous plaques, arterial calcification, and arteriosclerotic lesions developed along with renal disorder [47, 48]. Arteriosclerotic lesions were improved at low doses of calcitriol or paricalcitol administered to these mice, but aggravated at high doses. Therefore, it was suggested that active vitamin D might exhibit dual effects for arteriosclerotic lesions dependent on its concentrations [49]. Both lipid metabolism and inflammatory reactions are significantly involved in the formation of atheromatous plaques. Active vitamin D exhibits anti-inflammatory effects [50, 51], and may thus be involved in the prevention and improvement of atherosclerosis when dosed appropriately.

In the clinical setting, ultrasound examinations of the carotid artery in patients with hypertension and normal renal function showed that there was a negative correlation between the blood concentrations of $1,25(OH)_2D$ and intima-media wall thickness (IMT), suggesting a link between the vitamin D system and atherosclerosis [52]. During the past few years, numerous studies have been conducted in patients with chronic kidney disease (CKD) who exhibit a breakdown in the vitamin D metabolism pathway due to renal dysfunction. Since the major cause of death in CKD patients is cardiovascular complications, the role of the vitamin D system on cardiovascular function has been actively examined. In dialysis patients, the blood concentration of $25(OH)D$ or $1,25(OH)_2D$ is negatively correlated with the pulse wave velocity (PWV), but positively correlated with flow-mediated dilation (FMD) [53], suggesting a link between the vitamin D system and arteriosclerosis or vascular endothelial function.

Currently calcitriol and its analogs are routinely used for managing secondary hyperparathyroidism in CKD. The noted side effect of this class of drugs is hypercalcemia. Since hyperphosphatemia and hypercalcemia are known to contribute to the progression of vascular calcification in CKD patients, usage of active vitamin D has been linked to vascular calcification. In addition, some vitamin D analogs tend to over-suppress PTH. Excessive inhibition of PTH may damage the mineral buffering ability of bone, leading to surplus minerals in the blood which then promote vascular calcification. The effects of active vitamin D on vascular calcification are likely due to hypercalcemia since the direct effects of vitamin D analogs on vascular calcification have not been confirmed. On the other hand, low blood concentrations of $25(OH)D$ [54] and $1,25(OH)_2D$ [55] in CKD patients are associated not only with atherosclerosis but also with increased vascular calcification. Since VDR [56, 57] and CYP27B1 [36] are expressed in vascular smooth muscle cells, defective vitamin D - VDR axis in local blood vessel walls may contribute to the progression of vascular calcification. Furthermore, it has also been reported that usage of vitamin D analogs in CKD patients has nothing to do with the progression of vascular calcification [58]. Thus, the role of vitamin D analogs in vascular calcification in CKD remains to be clarified.

It is well recognized that left ventricular hypertrophy (LVH) is an independent risk factor of cardiovascular complications in CKD [59-61]. Pressure and volume overload, which increase with the progression of CKD, may cause necrosis of cardiomyocytes and the accumulation of fibrotic myocardial tissues, leading to LVH and decreased cardiac function. In the progression of LVH, many factors such as growth factor, nerve hormone, and cytokines may be involved [62-65]. It has been reported that administration of calcitriol improved LVH in dialysis patients [66, 67]. Paricalcitol, a vitamin D analog, improved ventricular diastolic capacity and left ventricular wall thickening in dialysis patients who received paricalcitol for at least 1 month (average administration period: 4.3 months; average dosage: 13 µg/week) during a 12-month observation period [68]. It was also reported that the blood concentrations of FGF-23, a newly identified regulator of serum phosphate and calcitriol levels, were linked to LVH in a calcitriol-independent manner [69]. More studies are needed to investigate how FGF-23 interacts with vitamin D analogs to regulate LVH. Additional information on FGF-23 is provided in subsequent chapters (see Chapters 4 and 7).

CONCLUSIONS

Approximately 40 years have passed since the discovery of calcitriol. However, the vitamin D field continues to progress. Our understanding of the vitamin D -VDR axis has advanced significantly because of the continuous efforts of researchers in conducting both preclinical and clinical studies. With our increased understanding of the multiple actions of the vitamin D -VDR axis, development of new agents to modulate VDR for the treatment of various diseases can be expected.

REFERENCES

[1]   Lawson DE, Fraser DR, Kodicek E, Morris HR, Williams DH. Identification of 1,25-dihydroxycholecalciferol, a new kidney hormone controlling calcium metabolism. Nature 1971; 230:228-230.

[2]   Holick MF, Schnoes HK, DeLuca HF, Suda T, Cousins RJ. Isolation and identification of 1,25-dihydroxycholecalciferol. A metabolite of vitamin D active in intestine. Biochemistry 1971; 10:2799-2804.

[3]   Baker AR, McDonnell DP, Hughes M, *et al.* Cloning and expression of full-length cDNA encoding human vitamin D receptor. Proc Natl Acad Sci U S A 1988; 85:3294-3298.

[4]   Malloy PJ, Pike JW, Feldman D. The vitamin D receptor and the syndrome of hereditary 1,25-dihydroxyvitamin D-resistant rickets. Endocr Rev 1999; 20:156-188.

[5]   Yoshizawa T, Handa Y, Uematsu Y, *et al.* Mice lacking the vitamin D receptor exhibit impaired bone formation, uterine hypoplasia and growth retardation after weaning. Nat Genet 1997; 16:391-396.

[6]   Li YC, Pirro AE, Amling M, *et al.* Targeted ablation of the vitamin D receptor: an animal model of vitamin D-dependent rickets type II with alopecia. Proc Natl Acad Sci U S A 1997; 94:9831-9835.

[7]   Takeyama K, Kitanaka S, Sato T, Kobori M, Yanagisawa J, Kato S. 25-Hydroxyvitamin D3 1alpha-hydroxylase and vitamin D synthesis. Science 1997; 277:1827-1830.

[8]   DeLuca HF, Suda T. [Current progress in the study of vitamin D--discovery of active vitamin D]. Tanpakushitsu Kakusan Koso 1969; 14:1068-1073.

[9]   DeLuca HF. Modern views of vitamin D. J Med Soc N J 1981; 78:611-613.

[10]   DeLuca HF, Schnoes HK. Vitamin D: recent advances. Annu Rev Biochem 1983; 52:411-439.

[11]   Lund J, DeLuca HF. Biologically active metabolite of vitamin D3 from bone, liver, and blood serum. J Lipid Res 1966; 7:739-744.

[12]   Norman AW, Lund J, Deluca HF. Biologically Active Forms of Vitamin D3 in Kidney and Intestine. Arch Biochem Biophys 1964; 108:12-21.

[13]   Fraser DR, Kodicek E. Investigations on vitamin D esters synthesized rats. Detection and identification. Biochem J 1968; 106:485-490.

[14]   Neville PF, DeLuca HF. The synthesis of [1,2-3H]vitamin D3 and the tissue localization of a 0.25-mu-g (10 IU) dose per rat. Biochemistry 1966; 5:2201-2207.

[15]   Blunt JW, DeLuca HF, Schnoes HK. 25-hydroxycholecalciferol. A biologically active metabolite of vitamin D3. Biochemistry 1968; 7:3317-3322.

[16]   Suda T, DeLuca HF, Schnoes H, Blunt JW. 25-hydroxyergocalciferol: a biologically active metabolite of vitamin D2. Biochem Biophys Res Commun 1969; 35:182-185.

[17]   Blunt JW, Tanaka Y, DeLuca HF. Biological activity of 25-hydroxycholecalciferol, a metabolite of vitamin D3. Proc Natl Acad Sci U S A 1968; 61:1503-1506.

[18]   Lawson DE, Wilson PW, Kodicek E. Metabolism of vitamin D. A new cholecalciferol metabolite, involving loss of hydrogen at C-1, in chick intestinal nuclei. Biochem J 1969; 115:269-277.

[19]   DeLuca HF. Vitamin D: the vitamin and the hormone. Fed Proc 1974; 33:2211-2219.

[20]   Madhok TC, DeLuca HF. Characteristics of the rat liver microsomal enzyme system converting cholecalciferol into 25-hydroxycholecalciferol. Evidence for the participation of cytochrome p-450. Biochem J 1979; 184:491-499.

[21]   Bjorkhem I, Holmberg I, Oftebro H, Pedersen JI. Properties of a reconstituted vitamin D3 25-hydroxylase from rat liver mitochondria. J Biol Chem 1980; 255:5244-5249.

[22]   Bjorkhem I, Hansson R, Holmberg I, Wikvall K. 25-Hydroxylation of vitamin D3 by a reconstituted system from rat liver microsomes. Biochem Biophys Res Commun 1979; 90:615-622.

[23]   Guo YD, Strugnell S, Back DW, Jones G. Transfected human liver cytochrome P-450 hydroxylates vitamin D analogs at different side-chain positions. Proc Natl Acad Sci U S A 1993; 90:8668-8672.

[24]   Rosen H, Reshef A, Maeda N, *et al.* Markedly reduced bile acid synthesis but maintained levels of cholesterol and vitamin D metabolites in mice with disrupted sterol 27-hydroxylase gene. J Biol Chem 1998; 273:14805-14812.

[25]   DeLuca HF. Evolution of our understanding of vitamin D. Nutr Rev 2008; 66:S73-87.

[26]   St-Arnaud R, Messerlian S, Moir JM, Omdahl JL, Glorieux FH. The 25-hydroxyvitamin D 1-alpha-hydroxylase gene maps to the pseudovitamin D-deficiency rickets (PDDR) disease locus. J Bone Miner Res 1997; 12:1552-1559.

[27]   Shinki T, Shimada H, Wakino S, *et al.* Cloning and expression of rat 25-hydroxyvitamin D3-1alpha-hydroxylase cDNA. Proc Natl Acad Sci U S A 1997; 94:12920-12925.

[28]   Galante L, Colston KW, MacAuley SJ, MacIntyre I. Effect of calcitonin on vitamin D metabolism. Nature 1972; 238:271-273.

[29]   Galante L, Colston K, MacAuley S, MacIntyre I. Effect of parathyroid extract on vitamin-D metabolism. Lancet 1972; 1:985-988.

[30]   Kong XF, Zhu XH, Pei YL, Jackson DM, Holick MF. Molecular cloning, characterization, and promoter analysis of the human 25-hydroxyvitamin D3-1alpha-hydroxylase gene. Proc Natl Acad Sci U S A 1999; 96:6988-6993.

[31]   Murayama A, Takeyama K, Kitanaka S, *et al.* Positive and negative regulations of the renal 25-hydroxyvitamin D3 1alpha-hydroxylase gene by parathyroid hormone, calcitonin, and 1alpha,25(OH)2D3 in intact animals. Endocrinology 1999; 140:2224-2231.

[32]   Brenza HL, Kimmel-Jehan C, Jehan F, *et al.* Parathyroid hormone activation of the 25-hydroxyvitamin D3-1alpha-hydroxylase gene promoter. Proc Natl Acad Sci U S A 1998; 95:1387-1391.

[33]   Murayama A, Takeyama K, Kitanaka S, Kodera Y, Hosoya T, Kato S. The promoter of the human 25-hydroxyvitamin D3 1 alpha-hydroxylase gene confers positive and negative responsiveness to PTH, calcitonin, and 1 alpha,25(OH)2D3. Biochem Biophys Res Commun 1998; 249:11-16.

[34]   Murayama A, Kim MS, Yanagisawa J, Takeyama K, Kato S. Transrepression by a liganded nuclear receptor *via* a bHLH activator through co-regulator switching. EMBO J 2004; 23:1598-1608.

[35]   Fu GK, Portale AA, Miller WL. Complete structure of the human gene for the vitamin D 1alpha-hydroxylase, P450c1alpha. DNA Cell Biol 1997; 16:1499-1507.

[36]   Somjen D, Weisman Y, Kohen F, *et al.* 25-hydroxyvitamin D3-1alpha-hydroxylase is expressed in human vascular smooth muscle cells and is upregulated by parathyroid hormone and estrogenic compounds. Circulation 2005; 111:1666-1671.

[37]   Kitanaka S, Katsumata N, Tanae A, *et al.* A new compound heterozygous mutation in the 11 beta-hydroxysteroid dehydrogenase type 2 gene in a case of apparent mineralocorticoid excess. J Clin Endocrinol Metab 1997; 82:4054-4058.

[38]   Dardenne O, Prud'homme J, Hacking SA, Glorieux FH, St-Arnaud R. Correction of the abnormal mineral ion homeostasis with a high-calcium, high-phosphorus, high-lactose diet rescues the PDDR phenotype of mice deficient for the 25-hydroxyvitamin D-1alpha-hydroxylase (CYP27B1). Bone 2003; 32:332-340.

[39]   Amling M, Priemel M, Holzmann T, *et al.* Rescue of the skeletal phenotype of vitamin D receptor-ablated mice in the setting of normal mineral ion homeostasis: formal histomorphometric and biomechanical analyses. Endocrinology 1999; 140:4982-4987.

[40]   Resnick LM, Muller FB, Laragh JH. Calcium-regulating hormones in essential hypertension. Relation to plasma renin activity and sodium metabolism. Ann Intern Med 1986; 105:649-654.

[41]   Burgess ED, Hawkins RG, Watanabe M. Interaction of 1,25-dihydroxyvitamin D and plasma renin activity in high renin essential hypertension. Am J Hypertens 1990; 3:903-905.

[42]   Li YC, Kong J, Wei M, Chen ZF, Liu SQ, Cao LP. 1,25-Dihydroxyvitamin D(3) is a negative endocrine regulator of the renin-angiotensin system. J Clin Invest 2002; 110:229-238.

[43]   Yuan W, Pan W, Kong J, *et al.* 1,25-dihydroxyvitamin D3 suppresses renin gene transcription by blocking the activity of the cyclic AMP response element in the renin gene promoter. J Biol Chem 2007; 282:29821-29830.

[44]   Fryer RM, Rakestraw PA, Nakane M, *et al.* Differential inhibition of renin mRNA expression by paricalcitol and calcitriol in C57/BL6 mice. Nephron Physiol 2007; 106:p76-81.

[45]   Artaza JN, Mehrotra R, Norris KC. Vitamin D and the cardiovascular system. Clin J Am Soc Nephrol 2009; 4:1515-1522.

[46]   Husain K, Ferder L, Mizobuchi M, Finch J, Slatopolsky E. Combination therapy with paricalcitol and enalapril ameliorates cardiac oxidative injury in uremic rats. Am J Nephrol 2009; 29:465-472.

[47]   Towler DA, Bidder M, Latifi T, Coleman T, Semenkovich CF. Diet-induced diabetes activates an osteogenic gene regulatory program in the aortas of low density lipoprotein receptor-deficient mice. J Biol Chem 1998; 273:30427-30434.

[48]   Davies MR, Lund RJ, Hruska KA. BMP-7 is an efficacious treatment of vascular calcification in a murine model of atherosclerosis and chronic renal failure. J Am Soc Nephrol 2003; 14:1559-1567.

[49]   Mathew S, Lund RJ, Chaudhary LR, Geurs T, Hruska KA. Vitamin D receptor activators can protect against vascular calcification. J Am Soc Nephrol 2008; 19:1509-1519.

[50]   Equils O, Naiki Y, Shapiro AM, *et al.* 1,25-Dihydroxyvitamin D inhibits lipopolysaccharide-induced immune activation in human endothelial cells. Clin Exp Immunol 2006; 143:58-64.

[51]   Martinesi M, Bruni S, Stio M, Treves C. 1,25-Dihydroxyvitamin D3 inhibits tumor necrosis factor-alpha-induced adhesion molecule expression in endothelial cells. Cell Biol Int 2006; 30:365-375.

[52]   Reis JP, von Muhlen D, Michos ED, *et al.* Serum vitamin D, parathyroid hormone levels, and carotid atherosclerosis. Atherosclerosis 2009; 207:585-590.

[53]   London GM, Guerin AP, Verbeke FH, *et al.* Mineral metabolism and arterial functions in end-stage renal disease: potential role of 25-hydroxyvitamin D deficiency. J Am Soc Nephrol 2007; 18:613-620.

[54]   de Boer IH, Kestenbaum B, Shoben AB, Michos ED, Sarnak MJ, Siscovick DS. 25-hydroxyvitamin D levels inversely associate with risk for developing coronary artery calcification. J Am Soc Nephrol 2009; 20:1805-1812.

[55]   Shroff R, Egerton M, Bridel M, *et al.* A bimodal association of vitamin D levels and vascular disease in children on dialysis. J Am Soc Nephrol 2008; 19:1239-1246.

[56]   Rajasree S, Umashankar PR, Lal AV, Sarma PS, Kartha CC. 1,25-dihydroxyvitamin D3 receptor is upregulated in aortic smooth muscle cells during hypervitaminosis D. Life Sci 2002; 70:1777-1788.

[57]   Wu-Wong JR, Nakane M, Ma J, Ruan X, Kroeger PE. Effects of Vitamin D analogs on gene expression profiling in human coronary artery smooth muscle cells. Atherosclerosis 2006; 186:20-28.

[58]   Wolisi GO, Moe SM. The role of vitamin D in vascular calcification in chronic kidney disease. Semin Dial 2005; 18:307-314.

[59]   Foley RN, Parfrey PS, Harnett JD, Kent GM, Murray DC, Barre PE. The prognostic importance of left ventricular geometry in uremic cardiomyopathy. J Am Soc Nephrol 1995; 5:2024-2031.

[60]   Foley RN, Parfrey PS, Harnett JD, Kent GM, Murray DC, Barre PE. Impact of hypertension on cardiomyopathy, morbidity and mortality in end-stage renal disease. Kidney Int 1996; 49:1379-1385.

[61]   Silberberg JS, Barre PE, Prichard SS, Sniderman AD. Impact of left ventricular hypertrophy on survival in end-stage renal disease. Kidney Int 1989; 36:286-290.

[62]   Hunter JJ, Chien KR. Signaling pathways for cardiac hypertrophy and failure. N Engl J Med 1999; 341:1276-1283.

[63]   Zoccali C, Mallamaci F, Maas R, *et al.* Left ventricular hypertrophy, cardiac remodeling and asymmetric dimethylarginine (ADMA) in hemodialysis patients. Kidney Int 2002; 62:339-345.

[64]   Middleton RJ, Parfrey PS, Foley RN. Left ventricular hypertrophy in the renal patient. J Am Soc Nephrol 2001; 12:1079-1084.

[65]   Valdivielso JM, Cannata-Andia J, Coll B, Fernandez E. A new role for vitamin D receptor activation in chronic kidney disease. Am J Physiol Renal Physiol 2009; 297:F1502-1509.

[66]   Park CW, Oh YS, Shin YS, *et al.* Intravenous calcitriol regresses myocardial hypertrophy in hemodialysis patients with secondary hyperparathyroidism. Am J Kidney Dis 1999; 33:73-81.

[67]   Kim HW, Park CW, Shin YS, *et al.* Calcitriol regresses cardiac hypertrophy and QT dispersion in secondary hyperparathyroidism on hemodialysis. Nephron Clin Pract 2006; 102:c21-29.

[68]   Bodyak N, Ayus JC, Achinger S, *et al.* Activated vitamin D attenuates left ventricular abnormalities induced by dietary sodium in Dahl salt-sensitive animals. Proc Natl Acad Sci U S A 2007; 104:16810-16815.

[69]   Gutierrez OM, Januzzi JL, Isakova T, *et al.* Fibroblast growth factor 23 and left ventricular hypertrophy in chronic kidney disease. Circulation 2009; 119:2545-2552.

CHAPTER 2

How Does Vitamin D Work?

Petya Valcheva and Jose M. Valdivielso[*]

Laboratorio de Investigación Hospital Universitario Arnau de Vilanova, IRBLLEIDA. Rovira Roure 80, Lleida, Spain

Abstract: Vitamin D is a seco-steroid hormone that has long been known for its important role in regulating body levels of calcium and phosphorus, and in mineralization of the bone. In addition to its endocrine effects, vitamin D has important autocrine/paracrine roles. The last step in the activation of vitamin D, the hydroxylation on Carbon 1, takes place mainly in the kidney. However, extra-renal sites have been also found to exhibit 25-hydroxyvitamin D_3-1-α-hydroxylase activity. The hormonally active form of vitamin D ($1,25(OH)_2D_3$, or calcitriol) mediates its biological effects by binding to the vitamin D receptor, a nuclear receptor. After the receptor is activated by calcitriol or its analogs, the protein changes its tridimensional conformation, which leads to key processes in mediating its nuclear actions such as binding to specific DNA sites to modify the expression of target genes. Several steps take place in order to increase or decrease the transcription rate of a target gene. First, homodimerization of the vitamin D receptor or heterodimerization with the retinoid X receptor allows the complex to bind to DNA. Then, several proteins are recruited to the complex that either increase or decrease chromatin condensation, thus acting like co-represors or co-activators, respectively, finally decreasing or increasing the target gene transcription. The co-activators bind to several extra proteins that build a bridge to the basal transcriptional machinery. Therefore, little changes in the receptor's tridimensional structure elicited by different analogs can lead to differences in protein recruitment and in gene transactivation. Furthermore, differences in the cellular environment can yield different responses to the same analog. This characteristic of the nuclear receptors makes them good candidates as valuable therapeutic targets.

Keywords: Co-represors, co-activators, 1,25-dihydroxyvitamin D, DNA binding domain (DBD), gene transcription, ligand binding domain, 25(OH)D, parathyroid hormone (PTH), VDR, VDRE, vitamin D metabolism.

VITAMIN D METABOLISM

In the recent years, a number of basic and clinical studies point to the important role that vitamin D plays in various physiological and pathological processes throughout the body. Vitamin D is a fat soluble pre-hormone with seco-steroid nature which shows conformationally flexible structural characteristic [1]. Vitamin D in humans can be obtained from the diet (vegetal ergocalciferol, or vitamin D_2, and animal cholecalciferol, or vitamin D_3). Vitamin D enters the blood circulation as a chylomicron/liproprotein complex after intestinal absorption [2]. However, the main source of vitamin D is endogenously synthesized from the precursor molecule 7-dehydrocholesterol in the skin by photolytic action of the solar UVB light. Once pre-vitamin D_3 is formed, it undergoes a spontaneous temperature-dependent thermal isomerization to vitamin D_3, which is then transported into the circulation and binds to the vitamin D-binding protein (DBP). DBP drives vitamin D_3 subsequently to the liver and then to the kidney for bioactivation as well as carries away inactive metabolites for catabolism and excretion.

In the first activation step, vitamin D_3 is hydroxylated by the cytochrome P450 enzyme 25-hydroxylase (CYP27A1) to 25-hydroxyvitamin D_3 ($25(OH)D_3$) mainly in the liver, but also in the kidney, intestine, brain, lung, skin, prostate gland, blood vessels and macrophages [3]. This enzyme 25-hydroxylates both vitamin D_2 and D_3. This first hydroxylation is poorly regulated. That's why the level of $25(OH)D_3$ in serum

*Address correspondence to Jose M. Valdivielso: Laboratorio de Investigación Hospital Universitario Arnau de Vilanova, IRBLLEIDA. Rovira Roure 80, Lleida. Spain. E-mail: valdivielso@medicina.udl.es

increases in proportion to vitamin D_3 intake. Being the most abundant form, the $25(OH)D_3$ level is used as a marker for the vitamin D status. When $25(OH)D_3$ levels are at 10 - 20 ng/mL (or 25 - 50 mmol/L), it is considered as vitamin D insufficiency. A level below 10 ng/mL is accepted as vitamin D deficiency. Normal levels are between 30 and 100 ng/mL. Serum levels of $25(OH)D_3$ are low in many people of all ages who live at northern latitudes and lower altitude, especially in the winter [4].

In the second step, the biologically active hormone 1,25-dihydroxyvitamin D_3 ($1,25(OH)_2D_3$) is generated by the mitochondrial enzyme 25-hydroxyvitamin D_3 1-alpha-hydroxylase (CYP27B1, 1α-hydroxylase). Circulating levels of $1,25(OH)_2D_3$ are tightly regulated. CYP27B1 is a monooxygenase attached to the inner mitochondrial membrane, with a molecular mass of approximately 52 kDa. In order to exert its actions, this enzyme requires molecular oxygen and NADPH-reducing equivalents from a group of iron-sulfur proteins called ferredoxins. The affinity of CYP27B1 for $25(OH)D_3$ differs between species and tissues with Km values ranging from 1 to 16 μM [5]. The hydroxylation at Carbon 1 in the $25(OH)D_3$ molecule occurs mainly in the kidney. The expression of this enzyme is found in both the proximal (endocrine function) and distal convoluted tubules (autocrine/paracrine function) in the kidney, but it is also found in numerous other tissues, organs and cells (lung, brain, liver, intestine, bone, stomach, spleen, colon, thymus, lymph nodes, skin, placenta, monocytes, dendritic cells, vascular smooth muscle cells, endothelial cells, *etc.*) [6, 7]. However, in humans, these extra-renal sources of $1,25(OH)_2D_3$ are thought to contribute to circulating $1,25(OH)_2D_3$ levels only during pregnancy, in chronic renal failure (CRF), and in pathological conditions such as sarcoidosis, tuberculosis, granulomatous disorders, and rheumatoid arthritis. Nevertheless, local production of $1,25(OH)_2D_3$ could be important as an autocrine or paracrine regulator of certain cell functions.

Low levels of $1,25(OH)_2D_3$ can be found in conditions like CRF and pseudo–vitamin D–deficiency rickets (PDDR). However, the pathophysiology is different because in CRF the compromised renal mass reduces CYP27B1 activity, whereas in PDDR there is a hereditary defect in the gene that codes for the CYP27B1. Some of the factors that influence the expression of the enzyme are parathyroid hormone (PTH), calcitonin, interferon gamma, calcium, phosphorus, and the active form of vitamin D itself. $1,25(OH)_2D_3$ directly suppresses CYP27B1 expression by a feedback loop as well as by suppressing the synthesis and secretion of PTH, which is the primary trophic hormone that stimulates the CYP27B1 expression [5, 8].

Under conditions of adequate plasma Ca^{2+} levels, the 24-hydroxylation of both $25(OH)D_3$ and $1,25(OH)_2D_3$ occurs under the enzymatic activity of CYP24A1 (1,25-dihydroxyvitamin D_3 24-hydroxylase or 24-hydroxylase). The CYP24A1 is a mitochondrial enzyme (~53 kDa) and is very tightly regulated at the transcriptional level by the active form of vitamin D in almost all tissues where VDR expression could be found, thus making possible a negative feedback mechanism [9]. The Km of CYP24A1 for $25(OH)D_3$ ranges from 0.5 to 3 μM, but the preferred substrate for CYP24A1 is $1,25(OH)_2D_3$, with its Km values approximately 10-fold lower (0.1 - 0.25 μM), making the enzyme very important in controlling the ambient $1,25(OH)_2D_3$ levels. The 24,25-dihydroxyvitamin D ($24,25(OH)_2D_3$) is the major circulating dihydroxy metabolite and is believed to have some biological activity in the intramembranous bone formation and the early stages of the fracture repair [10]. 24,25-Dihydroxyvitamin D is also readily hydroxylated by CYP27B1, and is actually the preferred substrate compared with $25(OH)D_3$. However, due to the 10-fold higher concentration of $25(OH)D_3$, the rate of $1,25(OH)_2D_3$ synthesis is greater than that observed for 1,24,25-trihydroxyvitamin D_3 ($1,24,25(OH)_3D_3$) [5]. It is known that $1,25(OH)_2D_3$ can be rapidly metabolized either to $1,24,25(OH)_3D_3$ and then to calcitroic acid or to $25(OH)D_3$-lactone. The first pathway consists of five sequential steps - C24 hydroxylation, C24 ketonization (C24-oxo) and C23 hydroxylation (C23-OH/C24-oxo), followed by an oxidative reaction in which 24,25,26,27-tetranor-1-alpha,$23(OH)_2D_3$ is formed to be transformed in calcitroic acid, a water-soluble metabolite, which is filtered in the kidney and excreted in the urine. The other pathway involves C26 hydroxylation, C23 hydroxylation and lactonization to form (23S,25R)-$1,25(OH)_2D_3$-26,23-lactone [11]. Similar C23/C24 oxidation pathways exist for $24,25(OH)_2D_3$.

VITAMIN D RECEPTOR

There are two known proteins with structurally different ligand binding domains that could specifically bind to calcitriol, the biologically active form of vitamin D: vitamin D receptor (VDR) (Kd = 1.2 nM) and DBP (Kd = 60 nM) [12].

VDR is a member of the superfamily of nuclear trans-acting hormone receptors (which include thyroid receptor, progesterone receptor, estrogen receptor, androgen receptor and glucocorticoid receptor) that regulate gene expression in a ligand-dependent manner. VDR has nearly ubiquitous tissue distribution (kidney, bone, parathyroid gland, intestine, lymphocytes, macrophages, tumour cells, *etc.*). Biochemical and *in situ* immunocytochemical localization studies have shown that VDR is likely a nuclear protein, even in the unoccupied state [13]. Unliganded VDR in the nucleus is bound to a co-repressor related to the so called silencing mediator for retinoid and thyroid hormone receptors (SMRT). VDR–SMRT complex is linked to histone deacetylase that maintains chromatin in a repressed state, thus repressing the transcription of target genes [14]. Other studies reported that VDR may reside in the cytoplasm in the absence of VDR ligands and the binding of $1,25(OH)_2D_3$ or some of its analogs makes the VDR move from the cytoplasm into the nucleus [15].

Vitamin D also exerts some rapid responses that are incompatible with a genomic response involving gene transcription. Some authors believe that the initiation of the rapid cellular responses to calcitriol occurs through a putative plasma membrane-associated receptor (mVDR). Candidates for the mVDR have been suggested, including annexin II [16], the MARRS (membrane associated, rapid response steroid) binding protein [17] and the classical VDR or a slightly truncated form of VDR associated with caveolae [12]. It has been proposed that the conformation of the ligand (6-s-*cis versus* 6-s-*trans*) may be linked to either rapid or genomic response. The 6-s-*cis* configuration of the ligand favours activation of the non-genomic rapid response pathways, whereas the 6-s-*trans* preferentially mediates genomic responses [1]. However, numerous studies have confirmed that the presence of a functional VDR is necessary for both the genomic and the non-genomic rapid responses to the active vitamin D_3 metabolite [18].

The human VDR (hVDR) is a product of a single chromosomal gene which locates on chromosome 12. The gene is comprised of at least 14 exons and span approximately 75 kb [19] (Fig. **1**). The VDR promoter lacks a TATA box initiator, is GC-rich and possesses putative binding sites for a variety of transcription factors. Six exons (1A to 1F) reside in the 5′-noncoding region, and eight additional exons (exons 2–9) encode the structural component of the VDR. In the kidney, at least three VDR mRNA transcripts are produced, possibly by differential splicing of 5′-noncoding exons. Most of the variant transcripts produce the same classical VDR protein of 427 amino acids with a molecular mass of ~ 48 kDa. VDR expression is regulated at both transcriptional and posttranslational levels. Single-nucleotide polymorphisms (SNP) in the VDR locus can be used to predict the susceptibility to suffer several disorders like osteoporosis, cardiovascular diseases and different types of cancer [20]. The most frequently studied polymorphisms in the VDR gene are the restriction fragment length polymorphisms (RFLP) for *BsmI*, *ApaI* and *TaqI*, found in intron 8/exon 9 at the 3′- end of the gene, together with the *FokI* polymorphism in exon 2 and the *Cdx2* polymorphism in the promoter region of the gene [21].

As a nuclear receptor, VDR has several functional domains. Based upon sequence analysis of the nuclear VDR, a membrane-spanning domain is unlikely. In the amino terminus there is an A/B domain that is 20 amino acids long. The DNA-binding domain (DBD), termed also C domain, locates between amino acids 21 and 92. As with other nuclear receptors, all VDRs described to date possess a conserved DBD consisting of two zinc finger motifs (residues 24–90 in hVDR), an α-helix residing on the C-terminal side of each zinc finger, with helix A and helix B constituting the DNA-recognition and phosphate backbone binding helices, respectively. One unique feature in the DBD of VDR is the presence of a cluster of five basic amino acids in the intervening sequence between the two zinc fingers (residues 49–55). Another interesting finding is that the DBD possesses a site (Ser-51) for hVDR phosphorylation by protein kinase C (PKC). This posttranslational modification makes the receptor unable to bind DNA. The flexible linker region (hinge) locates approximately between amino acids 93 and 123, followed by the E- or ligand binding domain (LBD) between amino acids 124 and 427. Three regions of hVDR in closest proximity to the $1,25(OH)_2D_3$ LBD would extend approximately from residues 227 - 240, 268 - 316, and 396 - 422. The C-terminal LBD is a globular multifunctional domain. It is responsible for hormone binding, strong receptor dimerization and interaction with co-repressors and co-activators, which are critical for the regulation of transcriptional activities. The LBD is formed by 12 α-helical structures. The twelfth helix contains a transactivation function 2 (AF-2) domain which suffers conformational change upon ligand binding and the orientation of Helix 12 determine the state of the receptor (either silent or activated) [22].

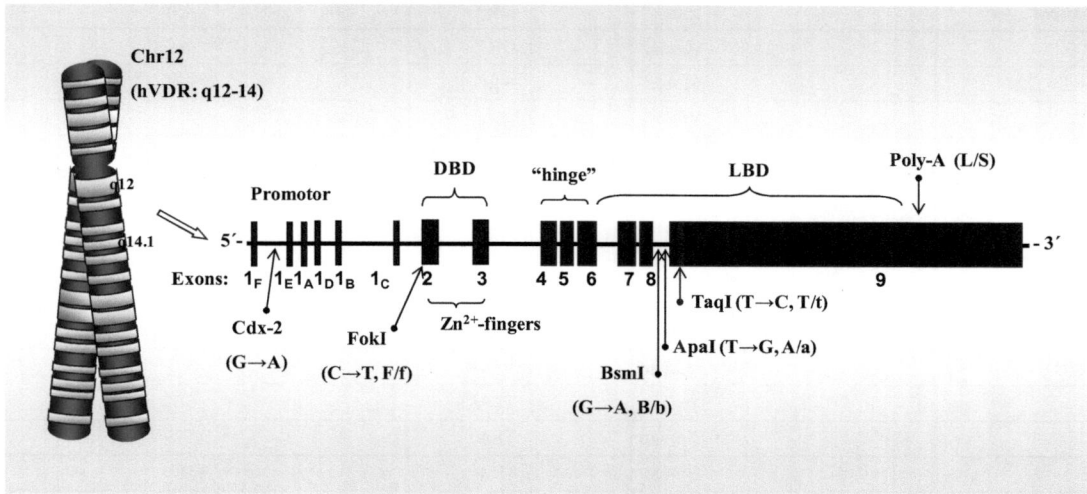

Figure 1: Schematic representation of the chromosomal localization and the domain organization of the human vitamin D receptor (hVDR) gene: DNA Binding Domain (DBD), "hinge" and Ligand Binding Domain (LBD), together with the positions of the five frequently studied single nucleotide polymorphism (SNP) sites.

The ligand-bound VDR can heterodimerize with retinoid X receptor (RXR) and then associate with specific genomic sequences in the promoter region of its target genes, known as vitamin D response elements (VDREs). However, some studies suggest that VDR represses some genes using a different co-partner other than RXR [23]. Several VDREs have been described in a variety of genes (Table **1**).

Table 1: List of some of the vitamin D responsive genes in normal and malignant cells

Gene	Species	Type of VDRE		References
CYP24A1	Human	DR3	(++)	[24]
Atrial natriuretic factor	Rat	DR3	(+)	[25]
Osteopontin	Mouse	DR3	(+)	[26]
Carbonic anhydrase II	Chicken	DR3	(+)	[27]
NPT2	Human	DR3	(+)	[28]
Osteocalcin	Rat	DR3	(+)	[29]
$p21^{Cip1}$	Human	DR3	(+)	[30]
Cyclin C	Human	DR3	(+)	[31]
Integrin β_3	Chicken	DR3	(+)	[32]
5-Lipoxygenase	Human	DR3	(+)	[33]
VEGF	Rat	DR3	(+)	[34]
PPARβ/δ	Human	DR3	(+)	[35]
IGFBP-3	Human	DR3	(+)	[36]
IGFBP-5	Human	DR3	(+)	[37]
TGFβ_2	Human	DR3	(+)	[38]
Insulin receptor	Human		(+)	[39]
RANKL	Mouse		(+)	[40]
PTH	Human	DR3	(-)	[41]
PTH related peptide	Rat	DR3	(-)	[42]
Growth hormone	Human	DR3	(-)	[43]

Table 1: cont....

RelB	Human	DR3	(-)	[44]
Type αI collagen	Rat	DR3	(-)	[45]
hTERT	Human	DR3	(-)	[46]
Calbindin D28k	Mouse	DR4	(+)	[47]
Pit-1	Rat	DR4	(+)	[48]
MYC	Human	DR4	(-)	[49]
Phospholipase C-γ1	Human	DR6	(+)	[50]
Fubronectin	Mouse	DR6	(+)	[51]
Calbindin D9k	Mouse	IP9	(+)	[52]
c-fos	Mouse	IP9	(+)	[53]
CYP3A4	Human	ER6	(+)	[54]
CYP27B1	Human	VDIR	(-)	[55]
Renin	Mouse	TFA		[56]
IL-2	Human	TFA		[57]
IL-12	Human	TRA		[58]
GM-CSF	Human	TFA		[59]

Note: The genes with described vitamin D response element (VDRE) are shown as positively (+) or negatively (-) regulated genes. The genes in which calcitriol regulates transcription by antagonizing other transcription factors are presented as TFA genes.

The typical response element found in the promoter region of the vitamin D responding genes has two hexameric half-sites with consensus sequence of RGKTCA (R = A or G, K = G or T). An example of a response element, formed by direct repeat of two hexameric core binding motifs spaced by three nucleotides (DR3-type) is the one found in the proximal promoter of the human CYP24A1. A VDRE with direct repeats spaced by four nucleotides (DR4-type) and six nucleotides (DR6-type) has also been described [60]. An additional important type of VDRE, the IP9-type, has an inverted palindromic structure with nine intervening nucleotides [61]. Another type of non-canonical VDRE is the everted repeat of hexanucleotide motif with a spacer of 6 base pairs (ER6 motif), described in the promoter region of human CYP3A4 gene [54], coding for one of the most important enzymes involved in the metabolism of xenobiotics in the body.

It has been shown that VDR binds to the 3′- half-site of the VDRE, while its heteropartner RXR interacts with the 5′- half-site [62]. Haussler *et al.* proposed that, in order to influence the gene expression of the target genes, VDR could reside on both the 3′- and the 5′- half-elements of the VDRE. Moreover, in the VDRE of positively regulated genes VDR is situated on the 3′- half-element, meanwhile in the VDRE of negatively regulated genes, VDR may have a reverse orientation, residing on the 5′- half-element [8].

MOLECULAR MECHANISM FOR VDR'S TRANSCRIPTIONAL ACTIVITIES

VDR can influence the expression of its responsive genes in two main ways: directly interacting with positive or negative VDREs in the promoter region and indirectly antagonizing the action of other transcription factors.

Ligand binding induces a conformational change in the VDR which initiates a series of events that promote the tight association of the receptor to its response element, enhance receptor dimerization, and generate new surfaces on the receptor. Those new surfaces allow the binding of co-activator molecules which are essential factors in the gene activation cascade [63]. Some authors suggest that ligand binding occurs in the cytoplasm whereas others propose that the union of the ligand to the receptor takes place in the nucleus. In any case, VDR activation induces VDR-RXR heterodimerization and recruitment of various co-regulatory molecules into the VDRE [64]. Numerous proteins and several protein-protein and protein-DNA interactions participate in a complicated chain of events.

Co-activators mediate induction of transcription, whereas the members of the family of co-repressors bind to the non-liganded VDR thus suppressing the expression of the target genes. The releasing of nucleosomal repression occurs through the replacement of the repressor by the co-activator complex, leading to the initiation of gene transcription [65]. Thus, in the un-liganded conformation histone deacetylases are recruited which deacetylate the lysine residues, resulting in chromatin compaction and silencing of genes. The $1,25(OH)_2D_3$ binding to VDR provokes conformational changes in Helix 12 of the LBD, making it closed and into the activation state. In this state the receptor promotes the dissociation of co-repressor molecules like the nuclear receptor co-repressor (NCoR) and Alien and the subsequent interaction of co-activators like the members of the p160 family (*e.g.* steroid receptor co-activator, SRC). The attachment of VDR-SRC or a VDR-histone acetyltransferase activity complex to a responsive promoter facilitates the destabilization of the nucleosomal core. These co-activator complexes probably act in a two-step process. First, a co-activator complex with histone acetyltransferase activity (CBP/p160) modifies chromatin and is then replaced by another co-activator complex (DRIP/TRAP) that interacts with RNA polymerase II. The unwound DNA then becomes a target for the VDR-DRIP (VDR-interacting proteins) complex, which contains mediator factors that are required for interaction with basal transcription factors and polymerase II [64, 66]. These protein complexes act as a direct link between the ligand activated receptor and RNA polymerase II holoenzyme complex and possibly recruit limiting components into the preinitiation complex. Multiple protein-protein interactions formed this way may enhance the stability of the complex and thereby facilitate the initiation of transcription [67]. In summary, in VDR mediated gene activation various co-activator complexes with distinct activities enter and exit their target promoter in an ordered manner and the action of one complex sets the stage for the arrival of the next one.

A few examples are presented here. In the CYP24A1 gene two VDREs are reported. In the absence of $1,25(OH)_2D_3$, the heterodimer VDR/RXR binds to one or both VDREs to recruit a co-repressor. Upon ligand binding to VDR, the co-repressor is replaced by a co-activator. When elevated levels of $1,25(OH)_2D_3$ (calcitriol) are present, both VDREs are used synergistically in order to induce high levels of CYP24A1, which in turn leads to efficient inactivation of the hormone. There are some factors like the PKC that could inhibit or enhance the $1,25(OH)_2D_3$ induction of CYP24A1 promoter activity [5].

In the promoter of parathyroid hormone (PTH) and PTH-related peptide (PTHrP) genes, VDR binds to a negative VDRE (nVDRE). This kind of VDRE is shown to be structurally different due to the fact that it contains a homologous sequence to only one of the two hexameric DNA sequences that form the VDRE for positive gene regulation by calcitriol [68]. In the case of the rat PTHrP two VDREs were reported by Falzon *et al.* to be responsible for the negative modulation of this gene [69]. A negative VDRE was also found in the CYP27B1gene promoter. However, a direct binding of VDR/RXR to this VDRE was not detected. In their study, Murayama *et al.* have shown that calcitriol suppressed the transcription of CYP27B1 *via* interaction with the bHLH-type transcription factor called VDR interacting repressor (VDIR). VDIR was found to be a direct sequence-specific activator of negative VDRE. The interaction between liganded VDR and VDIR induced the dissociation of p300 and association of histone deacetylase and co-repressors to directly mediate transcriptional repression [55].

One example for indirect regulation of gene expression is the negative action of calcitriol in the renin gene. Liganded VDR inhibits the binding of the nuclear cAMP response element-binding (CREB) protein to the cAMP response elements (CRE) located in the enhancer of the renin gene. This inhibition is by VDR's directly interacting with CREB in the ligand-binding domain, thus blocking the formation of CRE-CREB-CBP complex leading to reduction in renin gene expression [56]. Another example could be the suppression of the IL-2 expression after the inhibition of the formation of lymphoid cell-specific transcription factor NFAT-1/AP-1 transcriptional complex in the IL-2 gene promoter [57]. In a similar way, after the binding of $1,25(OH)_2D_3$, VDR represses the activated transcription of the granulocyte-macrophage colony-stimulating factor (GMCSF) gene. The interesting finding here is that VDR binds like a monomer in a different conformation from the one that is in the VDRE of positively regulated genes [59].

It has been shown that the transcriptional activity of VDR can be modulated in a positive and negative way in response to phosphorylation. Calcitriol itself has an essential role in this process activating different signalling pathways, including several kinases. For example, $1,25(OH)_2D_3$ provokes the translocation of the protein kinase C-β (PKC-β) to the nucleus and enhances its activity [70]. Furthermore, Hsieh at al. have shown that PKC-β plays a role in the control of VDR-mediated transcription, phosphorylating the hVDR in the region between the two zinc finger DNA-binding motifs (Ser-51) [71]. VDR is also a target of casein kinase II (CK-II), but in this case the phosphorylation of VDR is calcitriol-independent [72]. The phosphorylation at Ser-208 by CK-II leads to an increase in the transcriptional activation capacity of hVDR [73]. The phosphorylation in the region between the DBD and the LBD (at serine-182) in the hVDR has been shown to be achieved by protein kinase A and that this post-translational modification leads to an attenuation of both RXR heterodimerization and transactivation of $1,25(OH)_2D_3$ target genes [74].

OTHER PROTEINS THAT INTERACT WITH VITAMIN D METABOLITES

There are other factors in addition to VDR that are important for the regulation of the signalling pathways involving the vitamin D axis. Among them we can find the DBP and some proteins that promote internalization of steroid hormones, such as megalin (multiligand endocytosis receptor) and cubilin (endocytic glycoprotein receptor), both co-localized in the brush border of the renal proximal tubule epithelium [75]. Moreover, there is a group of hsp-70 related intracellular regulators called "co-integrator" chaperone proteins that guide the intracellular trafficking of vitamin D metabolites [76].

Even if assembled for maximal transcriptional effectiveness, the nuclear receptor transactivating complex must be able to interact with a specific promoter element in order to achieve its transcriptional potential. It has been shown the existence of a group of cis-acting proteins that compete with VDR-RXR for binding to VDRE, called VDRE-binding proteins (VDRE-BPs). These proteins belong to a family of more than 20 heterogeneous nuclear ribonucleoproteins (hnRNP-A, -B and -C) [77]. There are two important members, VDRE-BP1 (34-kDa) and VDRE-BP-2 (38-kDa), that exhibit different ability to remain on the cis element and interfere with VDR-RXR. It has been shown that in the absence of liganded VDR, the VDRE-BPs normally occupy VDREs and then the liganded VDR competes with VDRE-BP for binding to the proximal promoter of target genes. This relationship is disrupted when a natural elevation in VDRE-BP expression occurs as in the case of vitamin D-resistant New World primate cells [78].

VDR AGONISTS AND MOLECULAR BASIS FOR THEIR DIFFERENTIAL ACTIONS

The fact that the active metabolite of vitamin D, calcitriol or $1,25(OH)_2D_3$, exerts a variety of actions throughout the body, affecting different organs and systems, led to its identification as a potential therapeutic agent for the treatment of several disorders such as secondary hyperparathyroidism, osteoporosis, psoriasis, autoimmune diseases and different type of cancer (breast, prostate, colon). However, the therapy with calcitriol has some limitations because of the hypercalcemic and hyperphosphataemic properties of this agent, which may result in unwanted side effect like soft tissue calcification. In the past decades special attention has been paid to the development of structurally modified analogs of calcitriol as VDR activators or agonists (VDRAs) that are less hypercalcemic, but retain the beneficial properties [79]. Calcitriol ($1α,25(OH)_2D_3$) and VDRAs such as paricalcitol (19-nor-$1α,25(OH)_2D_2$) and doxercalciferol ($1α(OH)D_2$) are currently used to manage secondary hyperparathyroidism (SHPT) associated with CKD [80].

One of the differences among the different VDRAs is their affinity to DBP and other blood molecules like albumin and lipoproteins and VDR. Thus, VDRAs with higher affinity to DBP will stay longer in the circulation, whereas the ones with reduced affinity will be metabolized faster, reducing their availability [81]. Another difference is the ability of different cells to catabolise the compounds, regulating the levels of VDRAs in the cell [82]. Several structural modifications especially of the side chain such as fluorination or triple bonds markedly retard their catabolism mediated by CYP24A1 [83].

Furthermore, structure-function studies of the interaction between VDRAs and VDR reveal different binding modes in the ligand-binding pocket of the receptor [84]. Different pharmacophores in VDRAs may induce distinct AF2 conformational changes and cofactor interactions and can result in different modulation of receptor dimerization specific for different cell types [85], affect the DNA binding properties and even the promoter selectivity of VDR [60]. Thus, changes in ligand-receptor interaction may contribute to different biological actions [86]. For example, two of the VDRAs with changes at the side chain, AD47 and LAC67b, interact with the co-regulatory molecules in a differential way. AD47 induces the recruitment of the co-activator SRC-1 less efficiently than 1,25(OH)$_2$D$_3$, while LAC67b does not effectively recruit GRIP1 and ACTR, and also inhibits the interaction of these co-activators with VDR induced by 1,25(OH)$_2$D$_3$ [87].

Another mechanism to explain why different VDRAs have different effects is by the selective interaction of a transcriptional complex induced by a VDRA with a certain VDRE, since some variations in VDRE structures have been described. Quack *et al.* have shown that the transcriptional complex assembled upon VDR activation by the analog EB1089 has a higher affinity for DNA binding and a more sensitive (9-fold) activation of an IP9-type VDRE than of a DR3-type VDRE, whereas with the natural hormone calcitriol no VDRE preference could be observed [60]. Thus, different VDRAs can induce differential gene expression profiles in the same cell, resulting in what we call compound selectivity.

Furthermore, cellular environment can affect the response of a cell to a VDRA. Different cell types have different life-spans, from a short functional lifetime (intestinal cell) to a long-lasting active cell like osteoblast and parathyroid cell [88]. For example, the analog Ro-26-9228 induces significant interactions of GRIP and DRIP with the VDR in osteoblastic cells, whereas the same interactions are lower with VDR in intestinal CaCo-2 cells [89]. Thus, the same VDRA can induce different gene expression profiles in different tissues, resulting in what we call tissue selectivity.

Moreover, VDR activation creates an ubiquitination complex that leads to proteasomal degradation of VDR. Some of the most potent analogs (KH 1060, EB 1089) were found to retard the proteasome-mediated receptor degradation, thus enhancing their potency [86]. This may result in prolonged half-life of activated receptor and long-lasting effects in gene activation [90].

DIVERSE FUNCTIONS OF THE VITAMIN D-VDR AXIS

The metabolically active form of vitamin D, 1,25(OH)$_2$D$_3$ (calcitriol), regulates several functions in the body. It is now well accepted that 1,25(OH)$_2$D$_3$ regulates the calcium and phosphorus levels in blood *via* actions in the bone, parathyroid gland, kidney and intestine. Calcitriol is extremely potent in elevating serum calcium and phosphorus levels, and the concentration of the circulating 1,25(OH)$_2$D$_3$ is under tight regulation through its rates of synthesis and degradation. Major regulators of the 1,25(OH)$_2$D$_3$ concentration in the circulation are PTH, calcium, phosphorus and 1,25(OH)$_2$D$_3$ itself. More recently, numerous studies have demonstrate that 1,25(OH)$_2$D$_3$ is involved in several other biological responses (non-classical actions of vitamin D) that are not related to the control of mineral homeostasis.

Control of Mineral Homeostasis

Calcium levels are tightly regulated in order to support its roles in bone mineralization and cellular processes that include neuromuscular activity, intracellular signal transduction, and blood coagulation. The principal function of 1,25(OH)$_2$D$_3$, together with PTH, is to control the calcium and phosphorus status in order to ensure the availability of these minerals for biological functions as well as skeletal mineralization. This is achieved by coordinated actions of the parathyroid gland, kidney, intestine and bone. In addition, 1,25(OH)$_2$D$_3$ is also involved in regulating the synthesis of bone matrix proteins such as type I collagen, alkaline phosphatases, osteocalcin, osteopontin and matrix-Gla protein [91].

The most critical role of 1,25(OH)$_2$D$_3$ in mineral homeostasis is to enhance the efficiency of the small intestine to absorb dietary calcium and phosphorus, together with bone calcium and phosphorus resorption, and renal calcium and phosphate reabsorption, thus increasing the blood level of the Ca•PO$_4$ ion product. Intestinal calcium absorption occurs by both calcitriol–dependent active process in the ileum and passive diffusion process that can be positively affected by calcitriol. The active calcium absorption in the ileum relies on three primary components: epithelial calcium channels, intracellular calbindins and ATP-activated basolateral membrane calcium pump. It has been shown that $1,25(OH)_2D_3$ positively regulates the synthesis of these three components [92]. Thus, $1,25(OH)_2D_3$ increases the entry of calcium through the plasma membrane into the enterocytes and enhances the movement of calcium through the cytoplasm and across the basolateral membrane into the circulation. Furthermore, $1,25(OH)_2D_3$ is capable of reducing the excretion of calcium in the urine by increasing the reabsorption of calcium in the kidneys. Moreover, $1,25(OH)_2D_3$ is able to increase the mobilization of calcium from the bone into the circulation through the enhancement of osteoclastogenesis and osteoclastic activity. In relation to the ability of $1,25(OH)_2D_3$ to control the levels of phosphorus, one possible mechanism is the induction of phosphate translocating proteins in the kidney (renal sodium-phosphate cotransporter-2, NPT2) and probably in the small intestine as well. It has been shown that in hypophosphatemic conditions a stimulation of CYP27B1 occurs in order to produce adequate levels of $1,25(OH)_2D_3$. Then, $1,25(OH)_2D_3$ suppresses PTH levels and also induces both the phosphate-regulating gene with homologies to endopeptidases located on the X-chromosome (PEX) and the NPT2 genes. NPT2 has a direct effect over phosphate reabsorption in the kidney and the PEX enzyme can metabolize phosphatonins [8].

Pleiotropic Effects

Recently, it has been shown that VDR exerts its pleiotropic effects in a variety of target cells unrelated to its actions on mineral metabolism. For instance, VDR is shown to be involved in the regulation of vascular smooth muscle cell proliferation and calcification [93-95], in the regulation of the renin angiotensin system [96] and, in general, in cardiovascular health [97].

VDR regulates negatively the growth of breast, prostate and colon cancer cells. This effect may be related to the ability of the hormone-activated VDR to arrest the neoplastic cells in the G_1 phase of the cell cycle by influencing the regulatory proteins such as $p21^{Cip1}$ and $p27^{Kip1}$ [98], by controlling the proto-oncogenes such as c-*myc* and c-*fos* [52] or by down-regulating the *Bcl*-2 gene and inducing apoptosis [99].

It is known that VDR functions as a general suppressor of the immune system, including the activated B- and T-lymphocytes, especially the T-helper cells. Most immune cells express VDR as well as the enzymes responsible for its metabolism (CYP27B1 and CYP24A1). Dendritic cells are also targets of $1,25(OH)_2D_3$ in which it inhibits differentiation and maturation of these cells, leading to immunosuppressive activity [100]. In some *in vitro* experiments with dendritic cells, $1,25(OH)_2D_3$ treatment leads to down-regulated expression of the stimulatory molecules CD40, CD80, CD86 and the proinflamatory IL-12, and enhanced production of IL-10 that has potent anti-inflammatory properties. In addition, $1,25(OH)_2D_3$ inhibits the secretion of IL-2 by impairing the formation of the transcription factor complex NF-AT and IFN-γ through a VDRE mediated pathway [101].

There are some studies showing that $1,25(OH)_2D_3$ also affects several major endocrine processes, such as the TRH/TSH action and pancreatic insulin secretion, resulting in subsequent regulation of glucose homeostasis. VDR activation improves both insulin secretion and insulin sensitivity, which is associated with lower incidence of type II diabetes mellitus. This effect may be mediated by the presence of the VDR receptor and the CYP27B1 enzyme that catalyzes the formation of its active form in the pancreatic β-cells. VDR activation also influences the expression of the human insulin gene and insulin receptor and enhances insulin-mediated glucose transport *in vitro* [102].

$1,25(OH)_2D_3$ is likely to be an autocrine or paracrine factor for epidermal differentiation since it is produced by the keratinocyte. Keratinocytes contain VDR and all the enzymes required for the synthesis of $1,25(OH)_2D_3$ from 7-dehydrocholesterol. In keratinocytes $1,25(OH)_2D_3$, together with calcium, regulates the differentiation by turning on and off the genes and enzymes involved in the differentiation. It has been shown that during the differentiation of the keratinocytes VDR binds sequentially to two major co-activator complexes, DRIP (mainly the subunit DRIP205/TRAP220) and SRC, with a transition from DRIP in proliferating cells to SRC in differentiated cells [103]. The antiproliferative effects of vitamin D are accompanied by an increase in TGF-β [104] and a reduction in the number of high-affinity receptors for epidermal growth factor and the c-myc mRNA levels [105]. In addition, VDRKO mice show skin abnormalities such as dermal cysts, which were still present in mice fed a rescue diet, indicating that VDR plays a key role in regulating hair growth cycle and skin development, independent of its effects on the mineral homeostasis.

The anti-oxidative effects of vitamin D have been suggested by epidemiological and *in vitro* and *in vivo* laboratory studies. On one hand, it is likely that 7-dehydrocholesterol, both vitamin D_2 and vitamin D_3, and the metabolically active form, $1,25(OH)_2D_3$, are able to stabilize the membrane of normal cells against iron-dependent lipid peroxidation *via* an interaction between their hydrophobic rings and the saturated and unsaturated residues of the phospholipid fatty acid side chains, leading to decreased fluidity of the membrane [106]. In a recent study Bao *et al.* showed that $1,25(OH)_2D_3$ can protect non-malignant prostate cells from oxidative stress-induced cell death by reducing ROS-induced cellular injuries through transcriptional activation of glucose-6-phosphate dehydrogenase, a key antioxidant enzyme [107]. On the other hand, the antioxidant activity of vitamin D could also be due to the fact that $1,25(OH)_2D_3$ increases the activities of superoxide dismutase and catalase [108].

There are some studies which have shown that both vitamin D deficiency and excessive levels of vitamin D are associated with accelerated aging [109]. However, it has been also described that higher vitamin D concentrations are associated with a longer leukocyte telomere length, which may be linked to the potentially beneficial effects of this hormone on aging and age-related diseases [110].

Clinical and experimental data have also shown that VDR regulates some physiological brain functions. It has been shown that $1,25(OH)_2D_3$ is able to induce the expression of some neurotrophic hormones like glial cell-derived neurotrophic factor (GDNF), leukemia inhibitory factor (LIF), neurotrophin-3 and nerve growth factor (NGF), and may be important for neuroprotection, regulation of behaviour, antiepileptic effects and normal motor functions [8].

CONCLUSIONS

The vitamin D axis is a ubiquitous system with important actions in many cell types. The versatility of the receptor, together with continuous, active research in developing new VDRAs, has provided opportunities to utilize specific ligands to activate VDR in a very specific manner. However, many questions remain unanswered regarding the molecular mechanisms that follow VDR activation by ligand binding. Further research is encouraged in this exciting area that could yield important therapeutic improvements in the short term.

REFERENCES

[1]   Norman AW, Song X, Zanello L, *et al.* Rapid and genomic biological responses are mediated by different shapes of the agonist steroid hormone, 1alpha,25(OH)2vitamin D3. Steroids 1999; 64: 120-8.

[2]   Bikle DD. Vitamin D regulated keratinocyte differentiation. J Cell Biochem 2004; 92: 436-44.

[3]   Ichikawa Y, Hiwatashi A, Nishii Y. Tissue and subcellular distributions of cholecalciferol 25-hydroxylase: cytochrome P-450D25-linked monooxygenase system. Comp Biochem Physiol B 1983; 75: 479-88.

[4]   Valdivielso JM, Coll B, Fernandez E. Vitamin D and the vasculature: can we teach an old drug new tricks? Expert Opin Ther Targets 2009; 13: 29-38.

[5]   Omdahl JL, Morris HA, May BK. Hydroxylase enzymes of the vitamin D pathway: expression, function, and regulation. Annu Rev Nutr 2002; 22: 139-66.

[6]   Hewison M, Zehnder D, Bland R, *et al.* 1alpha-Hydroxylase and the action of vitamin D. J Mol Endocrinol 2000; 25: 141-8.

[7]   Zehnder D, Bland R, Williams MC, *et al.* Extrarenal expression of 25-hydroxyvitamin d(3)-1 alpha-hydroxylase. J Clin Endocrinol Metab 2001; 86: 888-94.

[8]   Haussler MR, Whitfield GK, Haussler CA, *et al.* The nuclear vitamin D receptor: biological and molecular regulatory properties revealed. J Bone Miner Res 1998; 13: 325-49.

[9]   Townsend K, Evans KN, Campbell MJ, *et al.* Biological actions of extra-renal 25-hydroxyvitamin D-1alpha-hydroxylase and implications for chemoprevention and treatment. J Steroid Biochem Mol Biol 2005; 97: 103-9.

[10]   St-Arnaud R, Glorieux FH. 24,25-Dihydroxyvitamin D-active metabolite or inactive catabolite? Endocrinology 1998; 139: 3371-4.

[11]   Ishizuka S, Reichel H, Norman AW. Synthesis and biological activity of 1 alpha,23,25,26-tetrahydroxyvitamin D3. Arch Biochem Biophys 1987; 254: 188-95.

[12]   Huhtakangas JA, Olivera CJ, Bishop JE, *et al.* The vitamin D receptor is present in caveolae-enriched plasma membranes and binds 1 alpha,25(OH)2-vitamin D3 *in vivo* and *in vitro.* Mol Endocrinol 2004; 18: 2660-71.

[13]   Clemens TL, Garrett KP, Zhou XY, *et al.* Immunocytochemical localization of the 1,25-dihydroxyvitamin D3 receptor in target cells. Endocrinology 1988; 122: 1224-30.

[14]   Kim JY, Son YL, Lee YC. Involvement of SMRT corepressor in transcriptional repression by the vitamin D receptor. Mol Endocrinol 2009; 23: 251-64.

[15]   Barsony J, Pike JW, Deluca HF, *et al.* Immunocytology with microwave-fixed fibroblasts shows 1 alpha,25-dihydroxyvitamin D3-dependent rapid and estrogen-dependent slow reorganization of vitamin D receptors. J Cell Biol 1990; 111: 2385-95.

[16]   Baran DT, Quail JM, Ray R, *et al.* Annexin II is the membrane receptor that mediates the rapid actions of 1alpha,25-dihydroxyvitamin D(3). J Cell Biochem 2000; 78: 34-46.

[17]   Khanal RC, Nemere I. The ERp57/GRp58/1,25D3-MARRS receptor: multiple functional roles in diverse cell systems. Curr Med Chem 2007; 14: 1087-93.

[18]   Zanello LP, Norman AW. Rapid modulation of osteoblast ion channel responses by 1alpha,25(OH)2-vitamin D3 requires the presence of a functional vitamin D nuclear receptor. Proc Natl Acad Sci U S A 2004; 101: 1589-94.

[19]   Zmuda JM, Cauley JA, Ferrell RE. Molecular epidemiology of vitamin D receptor gene variants. Epidemiol Rev 2000; 22: 203-17.

[20]   Valdivielso JM, Fernandez E. Vitamin D receptor polymorphisms and diseases. Clin Chim Acta 2006; 371: 1-12.

[21]   Bid HK, Konwar R, Aggarwal CG, *et al.* Vitamin D receptor (FokI, BsmI and TaqI) gene polymorphisms and type 2 diabetes mellitus: a North Indian study. Indian J Med Sci 2009; 63: 187-94.

[22]   Herdick M, Carlberg C. Agonist-triggered modulation of the activated and silent state of the vitamin D(3) receptor by interaction with co-repressors and co-activators. J Mol Biol 2000; 304: 793-801.

[23]   Mackey SL, Heymont JL, Kronenberg HM, *et al.* Vitamin D receptor binding to the negative human parathyroid hormone vitamin D response element does not require the retinoid x receptor. Mol Endocrinol 1996; 10: 298-305.

[24]   Chen KS, Deluca HF. Cloning of the human 1 alpha,25-dihydroxyvitamin D-3 24-hydroxylase gene promoter and identification of two vitamin D-responsive elements. Biochim Biophys Acta 1995; 1263: 1-9.

[25]   Kahlen JP, Carlberg C. Functional characterization of a 1,25-dihydroxyvitamin D3 receptor binding site found in the rat atrial natriuretic factor promoter. Biochem Biophys Res Commun 1996; 218: 882-6.

[26]   van den Bemd GJ, Jhamai M, Staal A, *et al.* A central dinucleotide within vitamin D response elements modulates DNA binding and transactivation by the vitamin D receptor in cellular response to natural and synthetic ligands. J Biol Chem 2002; 277: 14539-46.

[27]   Quelo I, Kahlen JP, Rascle A, *et al.* Identification and characterization of a vitamin D3 response element of chicken carbonic anhydrase-II. DNA Cell Biol 1994; 13: 1181-7.

[28]   Taketani Y, Miyamoto K, Tanaka K, *et al.* Gene structure and functional analysis of the human Na+/phosphate co-transporter. Biochem J 1997; 324 (Pt 3): 927-34.

[29]   Staal A, Van Wijnen AJ, Desai RK, *et al.* Antagonistic effects of transforming growth factor-beta on vitamin D3 enhancement of osteocalcin and osteopontin transcription: reduced interactions of vitamin D receptor/retinoid X receptor complexes with vitamin E response elements. Endocrinology 1996; 137: 2001-11.

[30]   Liu M, Lee MH, Cohen M, *et al.* Transcriptional activation of the Cdk inhibitor p21 by vitamin D3 leads to the induced differentiation of the myelomonocytic cell line U937. Genes Dev 1996; 10: 142-53.

[31]   Sinkkonen L, Malinen M, Saavalainen K, *et al.* Regulation of the human cyclin C gene *via* multiple vitamin D3-responsive regions in its promoter. Nucleic Acids Res 2005; 33: 2440-51.

[32]   Cao X, Ross FP, Zhang L, *et al.* Cloning of the promoter for the avian integrin beta 3 subunit gene and its regulation by 1,25-dihydroxyvitamin D3. J Biol Chem 1993; 268: 27371-80.

[33]   Seuter S, Vaisanen S, Radmark O, *et al.* Functional characterization of vitamin D responding regions in the human 5-Lipoxygenase gene. Biochim Biophys Acta 2007; 1771: 864-72.

[34]   Cardus A, Panizo S, Encinas M, *et al.* 1,25-dihydroxyvitamin D3 regulates VEGF production through a vitamin D response element in the VEGF promoter. Atherosclerosis 2009; 204: 85-9.

[35]   Dunlop TW, Vaisanen S, Frank C, *et al.* The human peroxisome proliferator-activated receptor delta gene is a primary target of 1alpha,25-dihydroxyvitamin D3 and its nuclear receptor. J Mol Biol 2005; 349: 248-60.

[36]   Peng L, Malloy PJ, Feldman D. Identification of a functional vitamin D response element in the human insulin-like growth factor binding protein-3 promoter. Mol Endocrinol 2004; 18: 1109-19.

[37]   Matilainen M, Malinen M, Saavalainen K, *et al.* Regulation of multiple insulin-like growth factor binding protein genes by 1alpha,25-dihydroxyvitamin D3. Nucleic Acids Res 2005; 33: 5521-32.

[38]   Wu Y, Craig TA, Lutz WH, *et al.* Identification of 1 alpha,25-dihydroxyvitamin D3 response elements in the human transforming growth factor beta 2 gene. Biochemistry 1999; 38: 2654-60.

[39]   Maestro B, Davila N, Carranza MC, *et al.* Identification of a Vitamin D response element in the human insulin receptor gene promoter. J Steroid Biochem Mol Biol 2003; 84: 223-30.

[40]   Kim S, Yamazaki M, Zella LA, *et al.* Multiple enhancer regions located at significant distances upstream of the transcriptional start site mediate RANKL gene expression in response to 1,25-dihydroxyvitamin D3. J Steroid Biochem Mol Biol 2007; 103: 430-4.

[41]   Kim MS, Fujiki R, Murayama A, *et al.* 1Alpha,25(OH)2D3-induced transrepression by vitamin D receptor through E-box-type elements in the human parathyroid hormone gene promoter. Mol Endocrinol 2007; 21: 334-42.

[42]   Kremer R, Sebag M, Champigny C, *et al.* Identification and characterization of 1,25-dihydroxyvitamin D3-responsive repressor sequences in the rat parathyroid hormone-related peptide gene. J Biol Chem 1996; 271: 16310-6.

[43]   Alonso M, Segura C, Dieguez C, *et al.* High-affinity binding sites to the vitamin D receptor DNA binding domain in the human growth hormone promoter. Biochem Biophys Res Commun 1998; 247: 882-7.

[44]   Dong X, Craig T, Xing N, *et al.* Direct transcriptional regulation of RelB by 1alpha,25-dihydroxyvitamin D3 and its analogs: physiologic and therapeutic implications for dendritic cell function. J Biol Chem 2003; 278: 49378-85.

[45]   Owen TA, Bortell R, Yocum SA, *et al.* Coordinate occupancy of AP-1 sites in the vitamin D-responsive and CCAAT box elements by Fos-Jun in the osteocalcin gene: model for phenotype suppression of transcription. Proc Natl Acad Sci U S A 1990; 87: 9990-4 .

[46]   Ikeda N, Uemura H, Ishiguro H, *et al.* Combination treatment with 1alpha,25-dihydroxyvitamin D3 and 9-cis-retinoic acid directly inhibits human telomerase reverse transcriptase transcription in prostate cancer cells. Mol Cancer Ther 2003; 2: 739-46.

[47]   Gill RK, Christakos S. Identification of sequence elements in mouse calbindin-D28k gene that confer 1,25-dihydroxyvitamin D3- and butyrate-inducible responses. Proc Natl Acad Sci U S A 1993; 90: 2984-8.

[48]   Rhodes SJ, Chen R, DiMattia GE, *et al.* A tissue-specific enhancer confers Pit-1-dependent morphogen inducibility and autoregulation on the pit-1 gene. Genes Dev 1993; 7: 913-32.

[49]   Toropainen S, Vaisanen S, Heikkinen S, *et al.* The down-regulation of the human MYC gene by the nuclear hormone 1alpha,25-dihydroxyvitamin D3 is associated with cycling of corepressors and histone deacetylases. J Mol Biol 2010; 400: 284-94.

[50]   Xie Z, Bikle DD. Cloning of the human phospholipase C-gamma1 promoter and identification of a DR6-type vitamin D-responsive element. J Biol Chem 1997; 272: 6573-7.

[51]   Polly P, Carlberg C, Eisman JA, *et al.* Identification of a vitamin D3 response element in the fibronectin gene that is bound by a vitamin D3 receptor homodimer. J Cell Biochem 1996; 60: 322-33.

[52]   Schrader M, Nayeri S, Kahlen JP, *et al.* Natural vitamin D3 response elements formed by inverted palindromes: polarity-directed ligand sensitivity of vitamin D3 receptor-retinoid X receptor heterodimer-mediated transactivation. Mol Cell Biol 1995; 15: 1154-61.

[53]   Schrader M, Kahlen JP, Carlberg C. Functional characterization of a novel type of 1 alpha,25-dihydroxyvitamin D3 response element identified in the mouse c-fos promoter. Biochem Biophys Res Commun 1997; 230: 646-51.

[54]   Thompson PD, Jurutka PW, Whitfield GK, *et al.* Liganded VDR induces CYP3A4 in small intestinal and colon cancer cells *via* DR3 and ER6 vitamin D responsive elements. Biochem Biophys Res Commun 2002; 299: 730-8.

[55]   Murayama A, Kim MS, Yanagisawa J, *et al.* Transrepression by a liganded nuclear receptor *via* a bHLH activator through co-regulator switching. EMBO J 2004; 23: 1598-608.

[56]   Yuan W, Pan W, Kong J, *et al.* 1,25-dihydroxyvitamin D3 suppresses renin gene transcription by blocking the activity of the cyclic AMP response element in the renin gene promoter. J Biol Chem 2007; 282: 29821-30.

[57]   Alroy I, Towers TL, Freedman LP. Transcriptional repression of the interleukin-2 gene by vitamin D3: direct inhibition of NFATp/AP-1 complex formation by a nuclear hormone receptor. Mol Cell Biol 1995; 15: 5789-99.

[58]   D'Ambrosio D, Cippitelli M, Cocciolo MG, *et al.* Inhibition of IL-12 production by 1,25-dihydroxyvitamin D3. Involvement of NF-kappaB downregulation in transcriptional repression of the p40 gene. J Clin Invest 1998; 101: 252-62.

[59] Towers TL, Freedman LP. Granulocyte-macrophage colony-stimulating factor gene transcription is directly repressed by the vitamin D3 receptor. Implications for allosteric influences on nuclear receptor structure and function by a DNA element. J Biol Chem 1998; 273: 10338-48.

[60] Quack M, Carlberg C. Selective recognition of vitamin D receptor conformations mediates promoter selectivity of vitamin D analogs. Mol Pharmacol 1999; 55: 1077-87.

[61] Carlberg C. Current understanding of the function of the nuclear vitamin D receptor in response to its natural and synthetic ligands. Recent Results Cancer Res 2003; 164: 29-42.

[62] Jin CH, Pike JW. Human vitamin D receptor-dependent transactivation in Saccharomyces cerevisiae requires retinoid X receptor. Mol Endocrinol 1996; 10: 196-205.

[63] Nolte RT, Wisely GB, Westin S, *et al.* Ligand binding and co-activator assembly of the peroxisome proliferator-activated receptor-gamma. Nature 1998; 395: 137-43.

[64] Nagpal S, Na S, Rathnachalam R. Noncalcemic actions of vitamin D receptor ligands. Endocr Rev 2005; 26: 662-87.

[65] Deeb KK, Trump DL, Johnson CS. Vitamin D signalling pathways in cancer: potential for anticancer therapeutics. Nat Rev Cancer 2007; 7: 684-700.

[66] Urnov FD, Wolffe AP. Chromatin remodeling and transcriptional activation: the cast (in order of appearance). Oncogene 2001; 20: 2991-3006.

[67] Chiba N, Suldan Z, Freedman LP, *et al.* Binding of liganded vitamin D receptor to the vitamin D receptor interacting protein coactivator complex induces interaction with RNA polymerase II holoenzyme. J Biol Chem 2000; 275: 10719-22.

[68] Nishishita T, Okazaki T, Ishikawa T, *et al.* A negative vitamin D response DNA element in the human parathyroid hormone-related peptide gene binds to vitamin D receptor along with Ku antigen to mediate negative gene regulation by vitamin D. J Biol Chem 1998; 273: 10901-7.

[69] Falzon M. DNA sequences in the rat parathyroid hormone-related peptide gene responsible for 1,25-dihydroxyvitamin D3-mediated transcriptional repression. Mol Endocrinol 1996; 10: 672-81.

[70] Simboli-Campbell M, Gagnon A, Franks DJ, *et al.* 1,25-Dihydroxyvitamin D3 translocates protein kinase C beta to nucleus and enhances plasma membrane association of protein kinase C alpha in renal epithelial cells. J Biol Chem 1994; 269: 3257-64.

[71] Hsieh JC, Jurutka PW, Galligan MA, *et al.* Human vitamin D receptor is selectively phosphorylated by protein kinase C on serine 51, a residue crucial to its trans-activation function. Proc Natl Acad Sci U S A 1991; 88: 9315-9.

[72] Jurutka PW, Hsieh JC, Haussler MR. Phosphorylation of the human 1,25-dihydroxyvitamin D3 receptor by cAMP-dependent protein kinase, *in vitro*, and in transfected COS-7 cells. Biochem Biophys Res Commun 1993; 191: 1089-96.

[73] Jurutka PW, Hsieh JC, MacDonald PN, *et al.* Phosphorylation of serine 208 in the human vitamin D receptor. The predominant amino acid phosphorylated by casein kinase II, *in vitro*, and identification as a significant phosphorylation site in intact cells. J Biol Chem 1993; 268: 6791-9.

[74] Hsieh JC, Dang HT, Galligan MA, *et al.* Phosphorylation of human vitamin D receptor serine-182 by PKA suppresses 1,25(OH)2D3-dependent transactivation. Biochem Biophys Res Commun 2004; 324: 801-9.

[75] Zhai XY, Nielsen R, Birn H, *et al.* Cubilin- and megalin-mediated uptake of albumin in cultured proximal tubule cells of opossum kidney. Kidney Int 2000; 58: 1523-33.

[76] Adams JS, Chen H, Chun RF, *et al.* Novel regulators of vitamin D action and metabolism: Lessons learned at the Los Angeles zoo. J Cell Biochem 2003; 88: 308-14.

[77] Chen H, Hewison M, Adams JS. Functional characterization of heterogeneous nuclear ribonuclear protein C1/C2 in vitamin D resistance: a novel response element-binding protein. J Biol Chem 2006; 281: 39114-20

[78] Chen H, Hu B, Allegretto EA, *et al.* The vitamin D response element-binding protein. A novel dominant-negative regulator of vitamin D-directed transactivation. J Biol Chem 2000; 275: 35557-64.

[79] Norman AW. The vitamin D Endocrine system: manipulation of structure-function relationships to provide opportunities for development of new cancer chemopreventive and immunosuppressive agents. J Cell Biochem Suppl 1995; 22: 218-25.

[80] Noonan W, Koch K, Nakane M, *et al.* Differential effects of vitamin D receptor activators on aortic calcification and pulse wave velocity in uraemic rats. Nephrol Dial Transplant 2008; 23: 3824-30.

[81] Brown AJ. Mechanisms for the selective actions of vitamin D analogues. Curr Pharm Des 2000; 6: 701-16.

[82] Brown AJ, Dusso A, Slatopolsky E. Vitamin D. Am J Physiol Renal Physiol 1999; 277: F157-F175.

[83] Eelen G, Valle N, Sato Y, *et al.* Superagonistic fluorinated vitamin D3 analogs stabilize helix 12 of the vitamin D receptor. Chem Biol 2008; 15: 1029-34.

[84]   Yamada S, Shimizu M, Yamamoto K. Structure-function relationships of vitamin D including ligand recognition by the vitamin D receptor. Med Res Rev 2003; 23: 89-115.

[85]   Liu YY, Nguyen C, Ali Gardezi SA, *et al.* Differential regulation of heterodimerization by 1alpha,25-dihydroxyvitamin D(3) and its 20-epi analog. Steroids 2001; 66: 203-12.

[86]   Jaaskelainen T, Ryhanen S, Mahonen A, *et al.* Mechanism of action of superactive vitamin D analogs through regulated receptor degradation. J Cell Biochem 2000; 76: 548-58.

[87]   Inaba Y, Yamamoto K, Yoshimoto N, *et al.* Vitamin D3 derivatives with adamantane or lactone ring side chains are cell type-selective vitamin D receptor modulators. Mol Pharmacol 2007; 71: 1298-311.

[88]   Bouillon R, Verlinden L, Eelen G, *et al.* Mechanisms for the selective action of Vitamin D analogs. J Steroid Biochem Mol Biol 2005; 97: 21-30.

[89]   Peleg S, Ismail A, Uskokovic MR, *et al.* Evidence for tissue- and cell-type selective activation of the vitamin D receptor by Ro-26-9228, a noncalcemic analog of vitamin D3. J Cell Biochem 2003; 88: 267-73.

[90]   Peleg S, Nguyen C, Woodard BT, *et al.* Differential use of transcription activation function 2 domain of the vitamin D receptor by 1,25-dihydroxyvitamin D3 and its A ring-modified analogs. Mol Endocrinol 1998; 12: 525-35.

[91]   White C, Gardiner E, Eisman J. Tissue specific and vitamin D responsive gene expression in bone. Mol Biol Rep 1998; 25: 45-61.

[92]   Wasserman RH. Vitamin D and the dual processes of intestinal calcium absorption. J Nutr 2004; 134: 3137-9.

[93]   Cardus A, Parisi E, Gallego C, *et al.* 1,25-Dihydroxyvitamin D3 stimulates vascular smooth muscle cell proliferation through a VEGF-mediated pathway. Kidney Int 2006; 69: 1377-84.

[94]   Cardus A, Panizo S, Encinas M, *et al.* 1,25-dihydroxyvitamin D3 regulates VEGF production through a vitamin D response element in the VEGF promoter. Atherosclerosis 2009; 204: 85-9.

[95]   Panizo S, Cardus A, Encinas M, *et al.* RANKL Increases Vascular Smooth Muscle Cell Calcification Through a RANK-BMP4-Dependent Pathway. Circulation Research 2009; 104: 1041-8.

[96]   Li YC, Kong J, Wei M, *et al.* 1,25-Dihydroxyvitamin D(3) is a negative endocrine regulator of the renin-angiotensin system. J Clin Invest 2002; 110: 229-38.

[97]   Valdivielso JM, Cannata-Andia J, Coll B, *et al.* A new role for vitamin D receptor activation in chronic kidney disease. Am J Physiol Renal Physiol 2009; 297: F1502-F1509.

[98]   Liu M, Iavarone A, Freedman LP. Transcriptional activation of the human p21(WAF1/CIP1) gene by retinoic acid receptor. Correlation with retinoid induction of U937 cell differentiation. J Biol Chem 1996; 271: 31723-8.

[99]   Kanli A, Savli H. Differential expression of 16 genes coding for cell cycle- and apoptosis-related proteins in vitamin D-induced differentiation of HL-60 cells. Exp Oncol 2007; 29: 314-6.

[100]   Penna G, Adorini L. 1 Alpha,25-dihydroxyvitamin D3 inhibits differentiation, maturation, activation, and survival of dendritic cells leading to impaired alloreactive T cell activation. J Immunol 2000; 164: 2405-11.

[101]   Adorini L, Penna G, Giarratana N, *et al.* Dendritic cells as key targets for immunomodulation by Vitamin D receptor ligands. J Steroid Biochem Mol Biol 2004; 89-90: 437-41.

[102]   Alvarez JA, Ashraf A. Role of vitamin d in insulin secretion and insulin sensitivity for glucose homeostasis. Int J Endocrinol 2010; 2010: 351385.

[103]   Hawker NP, Pennypacker SD, Chang SM, *et al.* Regulation of human epidermal keratinocyte differentiation by the vitamin D receptor and its coactivators DRIP205, SRC2, and SRC3. J Invest Dermatol 2007; 127: 874-80.

[104]   Kim HJ, Abdelkader N, Katz M, *et al.* 1,25-Dihydroxy-vitamin-D3 enhances antiproliferative effect and transcription of TGF-beta1 on human keratinocytes in culture. J Cell Physiol 1992; 151: 579-87.

[105]   Matsumoto K, Hashimoto K, Nishida Y, *et al.* Growth-inhibitory effects of 1,25-dihydroxyvitamin D3 on normal human keratinocytes cultured in serum-free medium. Biochem Biophys Res Commun 1990; 166: 916-23.

[106]   Wiseman H. Vitamin D is a membrane antioxidant. Ability to inhibit iron-dependent lipid peroxidation in liposomes compared to cholesterol, ergosterol and tamoxifen and relevance to anticancer action. FEBS Lett 1993; 326: 285-8.

[107]   Bao BY, Ting HJ, Hsu JW, *et al.* Protective role of 1 alpha, 25-dihydroxyvitamin D3 against oxidative stress in nonmalignant human prostate epithelial cells. Int J Cancer 2008; 122: 2699-706.

[108]   Sardar S, Chakraborty A, Chatterjee M. Comparative effectiveness of vitamin D3 and dietary vitamin E on peroxidation of lipids and enzymes of the hepatic antioxidant system in Sprague--Dawley rats. Int J Vitam Nutr Res 1996; 66: 39-45.

[109]   Razzaque MS, Lanske B. Hypervitaminosis D and premature aging: lessons learned from FGF-23 and Klotho mutant mice. Trends Mol Med 2006; 12: 298-305.

[110]   Richards JB, Valdes AM, Gardner JP, *et al.* Higher serum vitamin D concentrations are associated with longer leukocyte telomere length in women. Am J Clin Nutr 2007; 86: 1420-5.

CHAPTER 3

What Have We Learned from the Epidemiology of Vitamin D?

Csaba P. Kovesdy[*]

Division of Nephrology, Salem VA Medical Center, Salem, VA, Division of Nephrology, University of Virginia, Charlottesville, VA, USA

Abstract: Vitamin D deficiency has emerged as a potential risk factor for multiple adverse outcomes, including cardiovascular and cancer related morbidity and mortality. Epidemiological studies have been instrumental in detecting associations between lower serum levels of vitamin D and such outcomes, and by doing so have provided an impetus to examine the mechanisms of action underlying such associations and to design interventional trials of vitamin D supplementation to try and reverse the adverse effects attributed to low serum vitamin D. This chapter reviews in detail observational studies that describe the incidence and prevalence of hypovitaminosis D, and the various adverse outcomes that low serum vitamin D has been linked with. The comprehensive nature of this review will provide the reader with a better understanding of why vitamin D is currently regarded as a very promising area of research to try and lower adverse outcomes in a variety of patient groups and in the general population.

Keywords: All-cause mortality, cardiovascular risk factors, cardiovascular outcomes, cause-specific mortality, epidemiology, malignancies, hypovitaminosis D, National Health and Nutrition Examination Survey (NHANES), vitamin D supplementation.

INTRODUCTION

Vitamin D has captured the imagination of the medical community in the past decade. A deficiency in this "vitamin" that is not even a vitamin, but rather a hormone, has now been shown to be rampant in all segments of the general population and has been implicated in a variety of pathologic processes. But how did we learn about the roles of vitamin D in health and illness? All exploration starts with careful observations of the world around us, and the story of vitamin D is not different. Rickets, which is now known to be caused by vitamin D deficiency, became common during the industrial revolution as a result of the "modern" lifestyle of new city dwellers that resulted in significantly decreased exposure to sunlight. As early as in 1822 Jedrzej Sniadecki, a Polish physician working at the University of Wilno, recommended exposure to open air and sunshine for the cure of the "English disease" [1]. A similar link between lack of sun exposure and rickets was also observed by T.A. Palm in 1890 [2]. Subsequently the structure and the roles of vitamin D in the physiology of bone and mineral metabolism were elucidated. Interestingly, though, rather than relegating vitamin D and the consequences of its deficiency to the history books, scientists have been uncovering novel links between vitamin D deficiency and a variety of illnesses ever since. Epidemiologists have been at the forefront of such discoveries, as observational studies were instrumental in detecting both the extremely common nature of vitamin D deficiency and the associations that put the spotlight on the novel and complex roles of vitamin D. This chapter is focused mainly on the results of observational studies, but not on experimental data that in parallel with observational studies establish the biological plausibility underlying the link between low vitamin D levels and various morbid outcomes, nor on clinical trials that attempt to prove a cause-effect relationship between hypovitaminosis D and such outcomes. Throughout this chapter I will interchangeably use the terms serum vitamin D with serum levels of 25(OH)D.

PREVALENCE OF HYPOVITAMINOSIS D

Measurements of vitamin D levels have been performed in a large number of studies. A review by McKenna *et al.* [3] identified 117 studies that reported on serum levels of 25(OH)D between 1971 and

Address correspondence to Csaba P. Kovesdy: Division of Nephrology, Salem Veterans Affairs Medical Center, 1970 Roanoke Blvd., Salem, Virginia 24153, USA. E-mail: csaba.kovesdy@va.gov

J. Ruth Wu-Wong (Ed)

1990. These were in general small studies from various countries measuring 25(OH)D levels in the young or the elderly, and during various seasons. In healthy young adults 25(OH)D levels <10 ng/mL were almost never reported in North America [4-6], but were present in 4 - 9% of individuals in Scandinavia, with small seasonal variation [7, 8]. Interestingly, in other European countries the prevalence of such low 25(OH)D levels in young adults was >40% during winter months, but was almost non-existent during the summer [9, 10]; similar findings were reported from Saudi-Arabia [11, 12]. Similar to findings in healthy young individuals, healthy elderly persons also experience a high prevalence of low 25(OH)D levels during the winter, but a much lower prevalence during summer months, and more so in Europe [13-16] than in North America and Scandinavia [17-21]. Not surprisingly, studies examining institutionalized elderly persons have found significantly higher levels of severe hypovitaminosis D in these populations: levels <10 ng/mL were reported in up to 23% in North America [18, 22-24] and up to 100% in Europe [25-29]. Women tended to suffer from more severe hypovitaminosis D than men [20]. These studies have helped identify the major risk factors for hypovitaminosis D in the general population: season (less exposure to sunshine during winter months), latitude (less penetrating UVB radiation in countries at higher latitudes), nutritional deficiencies (more hypovitaminosis D in countries without fortification of foods with vitamin D or with dietary habits predisposing to less vitamin D intake), age (less skin production of vitamin D in the elderly) and mobility (less mobility predisposing to lower sun exposure especially in the debilitated and institutionalized elderly). Similar findings were reported in a number of more contemporary studies performed after 1990 [30-55]. In addition to the above listed risk factors of hypovitaminosis D race-ethnicity has also emerged as a risk factor [30, 31, 45], presumably because of the lesser ability to produce vitamin D in the integument of dark skinned individuals. Corroborating the above findings were some larger studies that started to emerge after the turn of the century. Lips *et al.* examined 7,564 premenopausal women who participated in an osteoporosis treatment study (Multiple Outcomes of Raloxifene Evaluation study), and found that 25(OH)D levels <10 ng/mL were present in 24% of the participating women [42]. This study also detected seasonal and geographic variations in 25(OH)D levels [42]. Hirani *et al.* [50] examined 1,766 participants in the Health Survey for England 2000 who were older than 65 years. Female gender, institutionalized status, poor health, lower socioeconomic status and low BMI were all associated with lower 25(OH)D levels in this study. Holick *et al.* [51] examined 1536 community-dwelling women and found 25(OH)D levels <20 ng/mL in 18%, <25 ng/mL in 36% and <30 ng/mL in 52% of them. Age, race, body mass index, vitamin D supplementation, exercise, education, and physician counseling were associated with vitamin D levels [51]. Brot *et al.* [55] examined 2,016 healthy middle aged perimenopausal females in Denmark and found that 7% of participants had 25(OH)D deficiency (serum levels <10 ng/mL) overall, but with significant seasonal fluctuation. In addition to the listed geographic, demographic and anthropometric characteristics chronic kidney disease (CKD) has also emerged as a comorbid condition associated with a significantly higher prevalence of hypovitaminosis D, possibly because uremia may adversely affect the photoproduction of cholecalciferol in the skin [56]. Wolf *et al.* [53] examined 825 incident hemodialysis patients and found that only 22% of patients had 25(OH)D levels >30 ng/mL; 60% of them had vitamin D levels of 10 - 30 ng/mL and 18% had levels <10 ng/mL. Seasonal variation in 25(OH)D levels was also present in this study, with blacks and diabetics displaying significantly lower serum levels. Levin *et al.* [57] examined 1,814 patients with various stages of CKD (non-dialysis dependent) and described median serum 25(OH)D levels of 20 - 30 ng/mL; levels were lower in patients with more advanced CKD, but without a statistically significant interaction between glomerular filtration rate (GFR) and 25(OH)D levels. It remains unclear if the lower 25(OH)D levels seen in patients with CKD and ESRD (end-stage renal disease) are related to a higher prevalence of conditions known to affect these levels (such as more black patients, more advanced age or a higher comorbidity burden with lesser mobility and sun exposure) *vs.* uremia-specific mechanisms leading to lower production, absorption and/or higher degradation of vitamin D.

A major advance occurred with the publication of studies from the National Health and Nutrition Examination Survey (NHANES), which allowed for a population-wide assessment of vitamin D status in the United States. Nesby-O'Dell *et al.* [45] examined 1,546 African American women and 1,426 white women who participated in NHANES III, and described a significantly higher prevalence of hypovitaminosis D (defined as levels ≤15 ng/mL) in non-Hispanic black compared to non-Hispanic white participants. Looker *et al.* [46] examined 18,875 NHANES III participants, finding 25(OH)D levels <7 ng/mL in <1%, <10 ng/mL in 1 - 5% and <25 ng/mL in 25 - 57% in subpopulations that were assessed either in the winter or at a higher latitude. The prevalence of hypovitaminosis D in the summer/higher latitude subpopulations was <1% - 3% for 25(OH)D <10 ng/mL and 21% - 49% for 25(OH)D <25 ng/mL. 25(OH)D levels were highest in non-Hispanic whites, intermediate in Mexican-Americans, and lowest in non-Hispanic blacks [46]. Zadshir *et al.* [52] reported data from 15,390 adult NHANES III participants and also found that ethnic minorities, the elderly and women had lower 25(OH)D levels. The population trends in 25(OH)D levels were illustrated by Ginde *et al.* [54], who compared 18,883 participants in NHANES III and 13,369 participants in NHANES 2001-2004. Mean 25(OH)D levels decreased from 30 (95% CI: 29 - 30) to 24 (95% CI: 23 - 25) ng/mL during the 10 years between these two phases of NHANES. The prevalence of 25(OH)D levels <10 ng/mL increased from 2% to 6% and those of >30 ng/mL decreased from 45% to 23% during these 10 years. The findings of this study underscore not only the high prevalence of low 25(OH)D levels, but also shed light on a worrisome trend of continuously worsening levels [54].

An important question arising from the studies examining the prevalence of 25(OH)D deficiency is the definition of "normal" 25(OH)D levels. Using values below 2 standard deviations of the normal population distribution of the 25(OH)D would clearly not be an accurate definition of "low" 25(OH)D levels, as these would represent levels that are much lower than those that have been established to signify important pathological bone and mineral metabolic processes [58]. An obvious deficiency in our knowledge is a lack of understanding of what thresholds to apply for complications of hypovitaminosis D that are unrelated to bone and mineral metabolism (discussed below). For the time being serum 25(OH)D levels >30 ng/mL are considered sufficient based on their impact on bone-mineral metabolism [58]. A significant proportion of the general population is thus suffering from abnormally low 25(OH)D levels, with certain subgroups being at a substantial disadvantage. The reason for this "epidemic" of hypovitaminosis D is unclear; a possible explanation is the continuing decrease in sun exposure brought about by a desire to lower the incidence of skin cancer. Furthermore, it remains unclear what to expect from population-wide interventions aimed toward correcting widespread hypovitaminosis D.

VITAMIN D AND CLINICAL OUTCOMES

While originally regarded as a regulator of bone and mineral metabolism, the functions of vitamin D are found to be far more diverse. Indeed, most cell types in the human body express vitamin D nuclear receptor, pointing towards biological functions unrelated to calcemic regulation. Some of these functions include down-regulation of hyperproliferative cell growth, immune modulation and down-regulation of the renin-angiotensin system [59-61]. The discovery of such wide-ranging effects has raised the possibility that the consequences of vitamin D deficiency could also be reaching far beyond those involving the skeletal system. Observations that individuals living at higher latitudes tend to suffer from higher rates of various chronic diseases such as cancers, hypertension or multiple sclerosis, and also experience higher mortality rates from certain types of malignancies, fuel speculations that the lower exposure to UVB radiation in these individuals with the resultant lower 25(OH)D levels might have accounted for the observed geographical differences in outcomes. It became necessary thus to examine if the lower 25(OH)D levels observed in so many individuals could be linked to poorer outcomes.

VITAMIN D AND ALL-CAUSE MORTALITY

All-cause and cause-specific mortality are the most important clinical outcomes; they also lend themselves as prime examination targets due to the certainty of the outcome and the availability of registries that allows the studying of large population groups. The first studies examining associations between serum 25(OH)D levels and mortality involved smaller samples drawn from single centers, secondary analyses of patients enrolled in clinical trials or special populations at high risk for adverse outcomes (which are easier to study due to the higher numbers of outcomes). Dobnig *et al.* [62] examined 3,258 adults undergoing coronary catheterization at a single medical center. Compared to the highest quartile, in the two lower quartiles of serum 25(OH)D levels the hazard ratio for all-cause mortality was 2.08 (95% CI: 1.60 - 2.70) and 1.53 (95% CI: 1.17 - 2.01). Another study exploring mortality associated with 25(OH)D levels was by Ng *et al.* [63] that examined 304 participants in the Nurses' Health Study and the Health Professionals Follow-Up

Study who were diagnosed with colorectal cancer. In this study the hazard ratio for all-cause mortality in the highest *vs.* lowest quartile of 25(OH)D was 0.52 (95% CI: 0.29 - 0.94), with a similar trend found for cancer-specific mortality. Two smaller studies examined survival associated with 25(OH)D levels in patients with non-small cell lung cancer. The study by Zhou *et al.* [64] examined overall and recurrence-free survival in 447 patients with early-stage non-small cell lung cancer and found that higher 25(OH)D levels were associated with better survival, especially in patients with stage IB-IIB cancers. A second study by Heist *et al.* [65] examined survival in 294 patients with advanced non-small cell lung cancer, finding no overall association of 25(OH)D levels with survival, albeit certain vitamin D receptor polymorphisms did show an association with better survival.

A number of studies examined outcomes associated with 25(OH)D levels in patients with CKD or ESRD, who are well known to suffer from a high prevalence of hypovitaminosis D and who are also experiencing extremely high rates of morbidity and mortality. Two of these examined patients with earlier stage, non-dialysis dependent CKD. Ravani *et al.* [66] studied 168 patients with non-dialysis dependent CKD who were enrolled at a single medical center over a two year time period. Lower 25(OH)D levels were significantly associated with higher all-cause mortality in this study. Another important finding of this study was that hypovitaminosis D was also associated with a higher incidence of end stage renal disease, raising the possibility that low 25(OH)D levels may also be involved in processes predisposing to progressive loss of kidney function. While of interest, this study was limited by the low number of participants and its single-center design, which limits our ability to generalize its findings. These drawbacks were offset in the study by Mehrotra *et al.* [67] that examined 3011 patients with non-dialysis dependent CKD from NHANES III, and found that individuals with 25(OH)D levels <15 ng/mL had an increased risk for all-cause mortality compared to those with levels >30 ng/mL, with a hazard ratio of 1.56 (95% CI: 1.12 - 2.18). The importance of this study is that its results are applicable to the entire non-institutionalized US population; its drawback is that there were few NHANES III participants who suffered from advanced non-dialysis dependent CKD, hence the results are mostly representative of patients with mild-moderate degrees of CKD. Patients on chronic dialysis were studied by Wolf *et al.* [53] who examined a prospective cohort of 825 incident hemodialysis patients and described significantly higher all-cause mortality rates in patients with lower 25(OH)D and 1,25(OH)$_2$D levels. Interestingly, the mortality risk imparted by lower 25(OH)D was mitigated by subsequent therapy with active vitamin D analogs in these patients, raising hopes that therapeutic interventions aimed at correcting the effects of 25(OH)D deficiency could successfully improve mortality. These findings reinforce the results of earlier pharmacoepidemiologic studies that have also indicated a lower risk of mortality in patients with CKD and ESRD treated with various forms of active vitamin D analogs [68-72]. However, due to the observational nature of these studies a cause-effect relationship between active vitamin D analog therapy and the improved outcomes cannot be ascertained, and the testing of this hypothesis would have to be done in randomized controlled trials.

The widespread presence of hypovitaminosis D in the general population (described in detail above) raises questions about the importance of this finding beyond patient groups that are at high risk for adverse outcomes, such as those with cardiovascular disease, CKD or cancer. The only study to examine all-cause mortality in a general-population based study was by Melamed *et al.* [73] This study included 13,331 adult NHANES III participants and found that those in the lowest *vs.* the highest quartile of serum 25(OH)D level (<17.8 *vs.* >32.1 ng/mL) experienced a 26% higher all-cause mortality (hazard ratio: 1.26, 95% CI: 1.08 - 1.46). The association of hypovitaminosis D with all-cause mortality was most pronounced in subgroups of participants without preexisting diabetes mellitus, cardiovascular disease or hypertension, suggesting that low 25(OH)D levels were not merely surrogate markers of underlying more severe morbid conditions, and allowing speculations that perhaps low 25(OH)D levels play an early role in the development of morbid conditions and subsequently in increased mortality [73]. Associations were also more pronounced in women, but the underlying mechanisms responsible for and the significance of this observation remain unclear.

The above studies provide compelling evidence implicating hypovitaminosis D as a risk factor of all cause mortality, but their observational nature renders such findings merely hypothesis-generating, and does not allow us to conclude that low vitamin D levels cause higher mortality. In order to do this one would have to show that interventions aimed at correcting low vitamin D levels can lower mortality. A meta-analysis of 18 randomized controlled trials of vitamin D supplementation showed that patients randomized to vitamin D supplementation experienced fewer deaths compared to those receiving placebo [74]. As the individual trials included in this meta-analysis have not always shown a significant effect of vitamin D supplementation, the clinical utility of such an approach remains unclear and requires further examination.

VITAMIN D AND CAUSE-SPECIFIC OUTCOMES

The association- between hypovitaminosis D and all-cause mortality poses questions about the mechanisms of action responsible for such associations. In order for hypovitaminosis D to be causally linked to overall higher death rates it is necessary to implicate hypovitaminosis D in morbid conditions that could than serve as intermediate steps toward the higher mortality. The plausibility of such links between hypovitaminosis D and various morbid conditions is supported by basic science data that link hypovitaminosis D to pathologic processes such as cardiomyocyte hypertrophy, excessive cell proliferation and renin-angiotensin system over-activation [61]. Several observational studies have examined associations of 25(OH)D levels with cause-specific mortality and with the incidence and prevalence of various morbid conditions. The most clinically relevant such conditions are cardiovascular disease and cancer, as these are responsible for most of the deaths observed in the developed world, and due to the larger number of outcomes these types of diseases lend themselves for examination in epidemiological studies.

Hypovitaminosis D and Cardiovascular Risk Factors

One plausible explanation for the higher all-cause mortality associated with hypovitaminosis D is that lower vitamin D levels may be associated with increased cardiovascular morbidity and mortality. Such a link could be due to a direct effect of hypovitaminosis D on vascular biology [75], but also due to an effect of various morbid states that are themselves known to be risk factors of cardiovascular disease.

An important risk factor for cardiovascular disease is hypertension. Due to the postulated link of vitamin D with blood pressure regulation [75] it is possible that low 25(OH)D levels can be causative of hypertension. Several ecologic studies have linked higher exposure to ultraviolet radiation to lower blood pressure [76-81], indirectly implicating vitamin D deficiency in hypertension. Building on these observations, and seeking a more direct link between vitamin D and hypertension were studies that examined associations between dietary vitamin D intake and incident hypertension. A small study that examined 86 women aged 20 - 35 yr and 222 women aged 55 - 80 yr reported a significant association between lower dietary intake of vitamin D and higher levels of systolic blood pressure [82]. Contrasting these earlier findings were the results of a study from Norway that included 7543 men and 8053 women aged 25 - 69, showing no association of dietary vitamin D intake with blood pressure levels [83]. These results were also echoed by a study that pooled data from 3 large and independent prospective cohorts (the Nurses Health Study I and II and the Health Professionals' Follow-up Study), where there was no association between the amount of dietary vitamin D intake and the risk of incident hypertension [84]. The reason for the lack of association between vitamin D intake and hypertension may have been the relatively small contribution of dietary vitamin D to serum 25(OH)D levels [85]. It is thus important to consider studies that examined the effect of directly measured serum 25(OH)D levels on blood pressure. Forman *et al.* [86] examined the association of measured 25(OH)D levels with incident hypertension in 613 men from the Health Professionals' Follow-Up Study and 1,198 women from the Nurses' Health Study, and of predicted 25(OH)D levels in 38,388 men and 77,531 women from the same cohorts. Both measured and predicted 25(OH)D levels showed a significant inverse association with the risk of incident hypertension in both men and women, indicating that a potential pathway for vitamin D to impact cardiovascular morbidity and mortality is through contributing to the development of hypertension. However, another population based study that examined 1,205 European individuals aged 65 years or older did not detect an association between 25(OH)D levels and systolic or diastolic blood pressure [87]. Such discrepancies will have to be resolved in future studies, including interventional trials.

Another important risk factor for cardiovascular diseases is diabetes mellitus. The link between vitamin D and diabetes mellitus was explored in several studies. In a report studying a group of Asian individuals from east-London Boucher *et al.* described a significant correlation between lower 25(OH)D levels and the presence of diabetes or impaired glucose tolerance [88]. Similar results were reported by Baynes *et al.* [89] who examined 142 elderly Dutchmen and described a significant association between low serum 25(OH)D levels and impaired glucose tolerance. Scragg *et al.* [90] examined 5,677 individuals in a cross sectional study and detected significantly lower 25(OH)D levels in those with new onset diabetes and impaired glucose tolerance. The same group of researchers examined 6228 individuals participating in NHANES III and again detected an inverse association between 25(OH)D levels and diabetes mellitus in non-Hispanic white and in Mexican-American participants, but not in non-Hispanic blacks [91]. The reason for the race-based differences is unclear; the authors speculated that it might reflect decreased sensitivity to vitamin D or to parathyroid hormone in blacks.

Seeking to explore the mechanism(s) underlying the association between vitamin D and diabetes, a study by Chiu *et al.* [92] examined the association of 25(OH)D levels with insulin sensitivity and beta cell function. Hypovitaminosis D was associated with both lower insulin sensitivity index and with higher glucose concentrations during an oral glucose tolerance test. These results support data obtained from animal studies indicating a direct effect of vitamin D on pancreatic beta cell function [93].

The association between 25(OH)D levels and a combination of various cardiovascular risk factors including hypertension and diabetes was also explored in a study by Martins *et al.* [94] which examined 7,186 males and 7,902 females from NHANES III. Patients with 25(OH)D levels in the first *vs.* the fourth quartile experienced increased odds ratios (OR) for hypertension (OR 1.30), diabetes mellitus (OR 1.98), obesity (OR 2.29), and elevated serum triglyceride levels (OR, 1.47, p <0.001 for all). Two other studies examined the association of 25(OH)D levels with the risk of metabolic syndrome in NHANES III participants [95, 96]. Both of these studies detected a significant association between lower 25(OH)D levels and increased odds of having the metabolic syndrome.

Together these studies support an association between hypovitaminosis D and various established risk factors of cardiovascular disease, suggesting a potential mechanism of action for how low 25(OH)D levels could be causing higher morbidity and mortality.

Hypovitaminosis D and Cardiovascular Disease

Cardiovascular diseases are the most important causes of mortality in the developed world, and vitamin D has been implicated in a host of functions directly related to vascular biology, atherosclerosis and blood pressure regulation [75], and also indirectly in the development of various risk factors of cardiovascular disease (see previous section). It is thus possible that vitamin D deficiency exerts its effects on survival through increased incidence and/or accelerated progression of cardiovascular pathology.

Cardiovascular mortality associated with 25(OH)D levels has been explored by numerous studies. In the study by Dobnig *et al.* [62] the hazard ratios for cardiovascular mortality in the two lower quartiles of serum 25(OH)D compared to the highest quartile were 2.22 (95% CI: 1.57 - 3.13) and 1.82 (95% CI: 1.29 - 2.58). Low serum 25(OH)D levels correlated with markers of increased inflammation, oxidative burden and cell adhesion in this study, supporting speculations that the mechanism of action for the observed association was indeed mediated through the various non-calcemic actions of vitamin D that directly affect the vasculature. Cardiovascular mortality associated with 25(OH)D levels was also examined by Pilz *et al.* [97] in this single center study 3,299 white patients referred for coronary angiography were followed for a median of 7.7 years. The hazard ratios (95%CI) for death due to heart failure and for sudden cardiac death were 2.84 (1.20 - 6.74) and 5.05 (2.13 - 11.97) in patients with 25(OH)D levels <25 nmol/L (<10 ng/mL) compared to persons with 25(OH)D ≥75 nmol/L (≥30 ng/mL). In a separate publication based on the same patient cohort lower 25(OH)D levels were also found to be associated with a higher risk of fatal strokes [98]. Mehrothra *et al.* [67] examined 3,011 patients with non-dialysis dependent CKD from NHANES III primarily for the risk of all-cause mortality associated with 25(OH)D levels, finding a significant inverse association, as discussed above. The risks for cause specific mortality (cardiovascular and non-cardiovascular) were also examined, and while these showed similar trends to all-cause mortality the associations were not statistically significant after adjustment for potential confounders. The lack of statistical significance could, however, be explained by the smaller sample size and the lower numbers of cause-specific events. Individuals with CKD on dialysis were examined by Wang *et al.*, who followed 230 peritoneal dialysis patients for 3 years or until death [99]. In this study every 1-unit increase in log-transformed serum 25(OH)D was associated with a 44% reduction in the hazard of fatal or nonfatal cardiovascular events (95% CI: 0.35 - 0.91; p = 0.018); this association was attenuated by subsequent adjustments. Last, but not least, cardiovascular mortality was one of the examined end points in the study by Melamed *et al.* [73] which utilized data from 13,331 adult NHANES III participants and described a significant association of low 25(OH)D levels with all-cause mortality. The association between 25(OH)D levels and cardiovascular mortality was similar to that seen for all-cause mortality, but statistical significance was not attained, perhaps due to the lower number of cause-specific events.

Numerous studies have explored associations between 25(OH)D levels and the incidence or prevalence of cardiovascular disease (CVD). The earliest studies were small case control studies which established associations with prevalent CVD, which were then followed by larger population based cohort studies examining incident events. In a case control study from 1978 Lund *et al.* [100] examined 128 patients hospitalized with ischemic heart disease and compared them to 409 control subjects, finding that 25(OH)D levels were lower in patients with angina or myocardial infarction. In a similar study from 1979 Vik *et al.* examined 30 cases with MI and 60 controls from northern Norway. This study detected no difference in 25(OH)D levels between cases and controls, but the small sample size made it difficult to interpret its findings. Scragg *et al.* [101] examined 179 patients from a single center who presented with myocardial infarction matched with controls by age and sex, and found a linearly decreasing risk of myocardial infarction associated with higher 25(OH)D levels. Small cross sectional studies have also established an association between lower 25(OH)D levels and increased severity of peripheral arterial disease [102, 103], with increased carotid artery intima-media thickness [104], and with increased severity of congestive heart failure [97]. Lower 25(OH)D levels were also associated with prevalent CVD in diabetic patients with chronic kidney disease, independent of the level of kidney function [105]. Associations have also been described between functional polymorphisms that determine vitamin D production and congestive heart failure [106]. The population-level associations between 25(OH)D levels and prevalent CVD were assessed by two studies that used data from NHANES. Kendrick *et al.* [107] studied 16,603 adult participants from NHANES III and described an increased prevalence of lower 25(OH)D levels in participants with underlying CVD; the adjusted odds ratio for prevalent CVD in those with 25(OH)D <20 ng/mL was 1.20 (95% CI: 1.01 - 1.36; p = 0.03). In the second study Melamed *et al.* [108] examined 4839 participants from NHANES 2001-2004, finding a linear decrease in the prevalence of peripheral arterial disease (defined as a low ankle-brachial index) across increasing quartiles of 25(OH)D levels. The multivariable-adjusted prevalence ratio of peripheral arterial disease in this study was 1.35 (95% CI: 1.15 - 1.59) for each 10 ng/mL lower 25(OH) D level.

The cross sectional design of the above studies did not allow for the assessment of incident CVD, which necessitates cohort study designs. De Boer *et al.* [109] investigated the associations of 25(OH)D levels with prevalent and incident coronary artery calcification in 1370 participants in the Multiethnic Study of Atherosclerosis (394 with and 976 without chronic kidney disease). Lower 25(OH)D levels were associated with incident, but not with prevalent coronary artery calcification; the association with incident coronary calcification was more pronounced in patients with chronic kidney disease. In another prospective cohort study of 18,225 men without preexisting CVD enrolled in the Health Professionals Follow-up Study Giovannucci *et al.* [110] described a significantly increased risk of myocardial infarction associated with lower 25(OH)D levels (relative risk, 95%CI: 2.09, 1.24 - 3.54 in persons with 25(OH)D levels <15 ng/mL *vs.* >30 ng/mL). In a similar cohort study based on 1,739 participants enrolled in the Framingham Offspring Study Wang *et al.* [111] described a significant increase in incident cardiovascular events in persons with lower baseline 25(OH)D levels (multivariable adjusted hazard ratio, 95% CI: 1.62, 1.11 - 2.36 in persons with 25(OH)D levels <15 *vs.* ≥15 ng/mL).

In summary, a large body of evidence links both incident and prevalent CVD to hypovitaminosis D. This link could be due to a direct effect of low vitamin D levels on vascular biology or due to the impact of hypovitaminosis D on more proximal causes of CVD such as hypertension or diabetes mellitus; alternatively, a combination of these could also be culpable for the observed effects.

Hypovitaminosis D and Malignancies

One of the multiple pleiotropic actions of vitamin D involves molecular effects that are important to prevent the initiation and progression of cancers, including the regulation of cell growth and the cell cycle, cellular differentiation and apoptosis [112, 113]. The possibility of a link between vitamin D and malignancies was, however, first raised by epidemiologists, long before the uncovering of the biologic underpinnings of such a relationship. As early as in 1941 Apperly observed that US residents living at higher altitudes experienced higher risk of death from common malignancies compared to people living in the Southern US States, and speculated that differences in exposure to sunlight might be responsible for this [114]. His observations went largely unnoticed until the latter decades of the past century when interest in vitamin D was revived and several other ecological studies have reexamined the link between various factors (such as geographical location, latitude or season) indirectly representing the amount of exposure to UVB radiation and mortality from various cancers. Studies examining the geographic distribution of colon [115], breast [116, 117], prostate [118] and ovarian [119] cancers have detected a significant negative association between lesser exposure to UVB radiation and increased mortality from these malignancies. Such ecological studies have started to proliferate significantly after the turn of the century, with the wider availability of registry data on the incidence and mortality of a large number of various malignancies from developed countries. The incidence and mortality of several malignancies has been consistently associated with decreased exposure to UVB radiation in virtually all of these studies, as recently reviewed by Grant and Mohr [120], strengthening the notion that vitamin D may have an important role in the development and outcome of cancers. The major limitation of these ecological studies is their lack of measurement of 25(OH)D levels; inferences can be made that a person living at a Northern latitude is probably exposed to less UVB radiation and hence probably has lower serum 25(OH)D levels, but it is likely that other environmental, cultural or socio-economic factors confound this association. It is thus important to examine if studies using actual measurements of serum 25(OH)D levels can corroborate the results of ecological analyses. Studying the association of 25(OH)D levels with specific types of cancers also poses additional analytical problems: event rates are in general lower which will lead to different methodologies compared to studies examining more common conditions, and the biology of distinct malignancies may be very different from each other and even the same type of malignancy can be heterogeneous depending on histological variants, which is why it is of interest to examine associations with different types of cancers separately.

Studies examining associations of 25(OH)D levels with overall cancer-related mortality have yielded less unanimous results compared to ecological studies. Giovannucci *et al.* [121] examined 47,800 men enrolled in the Health Professionals Follow-Up Study; of these, 4,286 developed incident cancers and 2,025 died from cancer-related causes after 14 years of follow-up. 25(OH)D levels were not measured in all participants, but were calculated using a regression model based on correlating measured 25(OH)D in a handful of participants with known predictors. In this study an increment of 25 nmol/L (10 ng/mL) in the predicted 25(OH)D levels was associated with a 17% reduction in total cancer incidence (multivariable adjusted relative risk: 0.83, 95% CI: 0.74 to 0.92), a 29% reduction in total cancer mortality (multivariable adjusted relative risk: 0.71, 95% CI: 0.60 to 0.83), and a 45% reduction in digestive-system cancer mortality (multivariable adjusted relative risk: 0.55, 95% CI: 0.41 to 0.74). Pilz *et al.* [122] examined the risk of fatal cancer in 3,299 patients from the Ludwigshafen Risk and Cardiovascular Health study and found that higher 25(OH)D levels were associated with lower risk of cancer-related mortality: the HR of the fourth 25(OH)D quartile was 0.45 (0.22 - 0.93) when compared with the first quartile and the HR per 25 nmol/L (10 ng/mL) higher 25(OH)D was 0.66 (0.49 - 0.89). Contrasting these two studies were two other studies that analyzed data from NHANES III. Freedman *et al.* [123] examined 16,818 participants in NHANES III and found that total cancer mortality was not associated with 25(OH)D levels; however, colorectal cancer-related mortality was inversely associated with 25(OH)D levels: 25(OH)D levels >80 nmol/L (>32 ng/mL) were associated with a 72% lower mortality. An inverse relationship was also found for female breast cancer related mortality, but the small number of outcomes related to this type of cancer limited the study's ability to reach robust conclusions. These results were echoed to some extent by Melamed *et al.* [73] in a study of 13,331 adults enrolled in NHANES III, in which all-cause mortality was significantly associated with lower 25(OH)D levels (as discussed above), but cardiovascular and cancer-related mortality did not show a significant association. The discrepancy between these studies could be explained by the heterogeneous outcomes associated with various different types of cancers, as it appears that associations between lower 25(OH)D levels and cancer-related mortality were robust for colorectal cancers, but may not be the same for other types.

It is hence of significant interest to examine how specific types of cancers associate with 25(OH)D levels. Most such studies did not examine cancer-related mortality, which would require large sample sizes and very long follow-up, but rather explored associations between 25(OH)D and the incidence of various cancers. Due to the lower number of the events of interest most such studies utilized a case-control design, often using data from large cohort studies (nested case control design). The link between colorectal cancers and 25(OH)D was strengthened by a study by Garland *et al.* [124] which examined 34 cases of colon cancer that were matched with 67 controls, drawn from data obtained in 25,620 volunteers in Washington County, Maryland who were followed from 1975 to 1983. The risk of colon cancer was reduced by 75% in the third quintile (27 - 32 ng/mL) and by 80% in the fourth quintile (33 - 41 ng/mL) of serum 25(OH)D, compared to the first quintile, and the risk of developing colon cancer decreased threefold in people with a serum 25(OH)D concentration of 20 ng/mL or more.

Studies examining associations between 25(OH)D and the incidence of other types of cancers, however, failed to find a similarly robust association. The risk of incident pancreatic cancer was examined by Skinner *et al.* [125] in the combined Health Professionals Follow-up Study and Nurses Health Study. A total of 365 cases of incident pancreatic cancer were diagnosed during the follow-up period of this cohort, and higher intakes of vitamin D were associated with lower risks for pancreatic cancer. Contrasting results were reported by Stolzenberg-Solomon *et al.* [126] who examined 200 incident pancreatic cancers matched with 400 controls in the Alpha-Tocopherol, Beta-Carotene Cancer Prevention cohort of male Finnish smokers, and found that higher 25(OH)D levels were in fact associated with higher odds of pancreatic cancer. The same group reanalyzed the risk of pancreatic cancer associated with 25(OH)D levels and this time found no significant association [127].

A large number of studies examined associations of 25(OH)D level with prostate cancer. With the exception of two Scandinavian studies [128, 129] none of these were able to detect a significant association between lower 25(OH)D levels and incident prostate cancer [130-136]; one study indicated that higher 25(OH)D levels were in fact associated with more aggressive histological types of prostate cancer [136]. Contradicting these latter results were findings by Li *et al.* [137] who examined 1,066 men with incident prostate cancer in the Physicians' Health Study that were matched to 1,618 controls and reported that 25(OH)D levels below the median were associated with increased risk of aggressive prostate cancer. The apparent contradiction between these two studies may have been explained by additional findings from Li *et al*, who also examined how the associations between 25(OH)D levels and prostate cancer were influenced by the genetic polymorphism of the vitamin D receptor: the presence of a less functional allele of the vitamin D receptor appeared to impart a significantly higher risk of aggressive prostate cancer in patients with lower 25(OH)D levels [137]. These latter findings again highlight the complexity of the biology of vitamin D, as genetic variants of its nuclear receptor can result in different biological activity and may explain why some of the earlier epidemiologic studies have reported discrepant findings. The importance of genetic variants in the vitamin D receptor were further highlighted by studies that found significant associations for certain types of polymorphisms - with prostate cancer [138-140] and with breast cancer [141].

Other explanations offered for the lack of association between 25(OH)D levels and non-digestive cancers (besides the genetic heterogeneity of the vitamin D receptor) included incidence-prevalence bias, confounding by lifestyle and sun exposure, misclassification bias, specific biological characteristics of certain cancer types (such as the loss of ability to convert 25(OH)D into $1,25(OH)_2D$ in prostate cancer cells) or the difficulty to ascertain relevant vitamin D status in the case of cancers that have long latency periods (such as prostate cancers) [142-144]. Due to such uncertainties it is paramount that the epidemiological studies are followed up by appropriately designed randomized controlled trials to test the hypothesis that vitamin D replacement could lower cancer incidence and mortality. The first large study that examined this hypothesis was the Women's' Health Initiative, which assigned 36,282 postmenopausal women randomly to receive 1,000 mg of calcium + 400 units of vitamin D *vs.* placebo, and examined among other endpoints the incidence of colorectal cancers [145]. Somewhat surprisingly there was no significant difference in colorectal cancer incidence between the intervention and the placebo arm, although the amount of vitamin D replacement may have been insufficient to have a major impact.

CONCLUSIONS

Vitamin D possesses very complex physiological functions and hypovitaminosis D appears to be involved in a host of processes related to the development and progression of multiple pathologic conditions. Epidemiologic studies have been instrumental in directing attention to the common nature of low 25(OH)D levels in the general population, and to the link between low 25(OH)D levels and important outcomes such as all-cause and cause specific mortality and morbidity. Due to the widespread nature of hypovitaminosis D the clinical implications of such links could be very significant. Inherent limitations of epidemiologic studies mandate that the observations made in such studies be followed up by prospective interventional studies to explore the effects of vitamin D supplementation on health and illness.

REFERENCES

[1]   Sniadecki J. In: Dziela. Warsaw: 1840: 273-274.

[2]   Harris LJ. Vitamins in Theory and Practice. In. Cambridge: 1935: 110.

[3]   McKenna MJ. Differences in vitamin D status between countries in young adults and the elderly. Am J Med 1992; 93:69-77.

[4]   Haddad JG, Jr., Hahn TJ. Natural and synthetic sources of circulating 25-hydroxyvitamin D in man. Nature 1973; 244:515-7.

[5]   Chesney RW, Rosen JF, Hamstra AJ, *et al.* Absence of seasonal variation in serum concentrations of 1,25-dihydroxyvitamin D despite a rise in 25-hydroxyvitamin D in summer. J Clin Endocrinol Metab 1981; 53:139-42.

[6]   Stryd RP, Gilbertson TJ, Brunden MN. A seasonal variation study of 25-hydroxyvitamin D3 serum levels in normal humans. J Clin Endocrinol Metab 1979; 48:771-5.

[7]   Lund B, Sorensen OH. Measurement of 25-hydroxyvitamin D in serum and its relation to sunshine, age and vitamin D intake in the Danish population. Scand J Clin Lab Invest 1979; 39:23-30.

[8]   Vik T, Try K, Stromme JH. The vitamin D status of man at 70 degrees north. Scand J Clin Lab Invest 1980; 40:227-32.

[9]   Murray B, Freaney R. Serum 25-hydroxy vitamin D in normal and osteomalacic subjects: a comparison of two assay techniques. Ir J Med Sci 1979; 148:15-9.

[10]   Preece MA, O'Riordan JL, Lawson DE, Kodicek E. A competitive protein-binding assay for 25-hydroxycholecalciferol and 25-hydroxyergocalciferol in serum. Clin Chim Acta 1974; 54:235-42.

[11]   Sedrani SH, Elidrissy AW, El Arabi KM. Sunlight and vitamin D status in normal Saudi subjects. Am J Clin Nutr 1983; 38:129-32.

[12]   Sedrani SH. Vitamin D status of Saudi men. Trop Geogr Med 1984; 36:181-7.

[13]   Bouillon RA, Auwerx JH, Lissens WD, Pelemans WK. Vitamin D status in the elderly: seasonal substrate deficiency causes 1,25-dihydroxycholecalciferol deficiency. Am J Clin Nutr 1987; 45:755-63.

[14]   Schmidt-Gayk H, Goossen J, Lendle F, Seidel D. Serum 25-hydroxycalciferol in myocardial infarction. Atherosclerosis 1977; 26:55-8.

[15]   Rapin CH, Lagier R, Boivin G, *et al.* Biochemical findings in blood of aged patients with femoral neck fractures: a contribution to the detection of occult osteomalacia. Calcif Tissue Int 1982; 34:465-9.

[16]   Stamp TC, Round JM. Seasonal changes in human plasma levels of 25-hydroxyvitamin D. Nature 1974; 247:563-5.

[17]   Delvin EE, Imbach A, Copti M. Vitamin D nutritional status and related biochemical indices in an autonomous elderly population. Am J Clin Nutr 1988; 48:373-8.

[18]   Clemens TL, Zhou XY, Myles M, *et al.* Serum vitamin D2 and vitamin D3 metabolite concentrations and absorption of vitamin D2 in elderly subjects. J Clin Endocrinol Metab 1986; 63:656-60.

[19]   Lukert BP, Carey M, McCarty B *et al.* Influence of nutritional factors on calciumregulating hormones and bone loss. Calcif Tissue Int 1987; 40:119-25.

[20]   Omdahl JL, Garry PJ, Hunsaker LA, *et al.* Nutritional status in a healthy elderly population: vitamin D. Am J Clin Nutr 1982; 36:1225-33.

[21]   von KJ, Slatis P, Weber TH, Helenius T. Serum levels of 25-hydroxyvitamin D, 24,25-dihydroxyvitamin D and parathyroid hormone in patients with femoral neck fracture in southern Finland. Clin Endocrinol (Oxf) 1982; 17:189-94.

[22]   Davies M, Mawer EB, Hann JT, Taylor JL. Seasonal changes in the biochemical indices of vitamin D deficiency in the elderly: a comparison of people in residential homes, long-stay wards and attending a day hospital. Age Ageing 1986; 15:77-83.

[23]   Dandona P, Menon RK, Shenoy R, *et al.* Low 1,25-dihydroxyvitamin D, secondary hyperparathyroidism, and normal osteocalcin in elderly subjects. J Clin Endocrinol Metab 1986; 63:459-62.

[24]   Rudman D, Rudman IW, Mattson DE, *et al.* Fractures in the men of a Veterans Administration Nursing Home: relation to 1,25-dihydroxyvitamin D. J Am Coll Nutr 1989; 8:324-34.

[25]   McKenna MJ, Freaney R, Meade A, Muldowney FP. Hypovitaminosis D and elevated serum alkaline phosphatase in elderly Irish people. Am J Clin Nutr 1985; 41:101-9.

[26]   Newton HM, Sheltawy M, Hay AW, Morgan B. The relations between vitamin D2 and D3 in the diet and plasma 25OHD2 and 25OHD3 in elderly women in Great Britain. Am J Clin Nutr 1985; 41:760-4.

[27]   Weisman Y, Salama R, Harell A, Edelstein S. Serum 24,25-dihydroxyvitamin D and 25-hydroxyvitamin D concentrations in femoral neck fracture. Br Med J 1978; 2:1196-7.

[28]   Preece MA, TomlinsonS, Ribot CA *et al.* Studies of vitamin D deficiency in man. Q J Med 1975; 44:575-89.

[29]   Corless D, Boucher BJ, Cohen RD, *et al.* Vitamin-D status in long-stay geriatric patients. Lancet 1975; 1:1404-6.

[30]   Harris SS, Dawson-Hughes B. Seasonal changes in plasma 25-hydroxyvitamin D concentrations of young American black and white women. Am J Clin Nutr 1998; 67:1232-6.

[31]   Harris SS, Soteriades E, Coolidge JA, *et al.* Vitamin D insufficiency and hyperparathyroidism in a low income, multiracial, elderly population. J Clin Endocrinol Metab 2000; 85:4125-30.

[32]   Lebrun JB, Moffatt ME, Mundy RJ *et al.* Vitamin D deficiency in a Manitoba community. Can J Public Health 1993; 84:394-6.

[33]   Gloth FM, III, Gundberg CM, Hollis BW, *et al.* Vitamin D deficiency in homebound elderly persons. JAMA 1995; 274:1683-6.

[34]   Chapuy MC, Preziosi P, Maamer M *et al.* Prevalence of vitamin D insufficiency in an adult normal population. Osteoporos Int 1997; 7:439-43.

[35]   Liu BA, Gordon M, Labranche JM, *et al.* Seasonal prevalence of vitamin D deficiency in institutionalized older adults. J Am Geriatr Soc 1997; 45:598-603.

[36]   Kinyamu HK, Gallagher JC, Rafferty KA, Balhorn KE. Dietary calcium and vitamin D intake in elderly women: effect on serum parathyroid hormone and vitamin D metabolites. Am J Clin Nutr 1998; 67:342-8.

[37]   Thomas MK, Lloyd-Jones DM, Thadhani RI *et al.* Hypovitaminosis D in medical inpatients. N Engl J Med 1998; 338:777-83.

[38]   Bettica P, Bevilacqua M, Vago T, Norbiato G. High prevalence of hypovitaminosis D among free-living postmenopausal women referred to an osteoporosis outpatient clinic in northern Italy for initial screening. Osteoporos Int 1999; 9:226-9.

[39]   Waiters B, Godel JC, Basu TK. Perinatal vitamin D and calcium status of northern Canadian mothers and their newborn infants. J Am Coll Nutr 1999; 18:122-6.

[40]   Outila TA, Karkkainen MU, Lamberg-Allardt CJ. Vitamin D status affects serum parathyroid hormone concentrations during winter in female adolescents: associations with forearm bone mineral density. Am J Clin Nutr 2001; 74:206-10.

[41]   Kauppinen-Makelin R, Tahtela R, Loyttyniemi E, *et al.* A high prevalence of hypovitaminosis D in Finnish medical in- and outpatients. J Intern Med 2001; 249:559-63.

[42]   Lips P, Duong T, Oleksik A *et al.* A global study of vitamin D status and parathyroid function in postmenopausal women with osteoporosis: baseline data from the multiple outcomes of raloxifene evaluation clinical trial. J Clin Endocrinol Metab 2001; 86:1212-21.

[43]   Vieth R, Cole DE, Hawker GA, *et al.* Wintertime vitamin D insufficiency is common in young Canadian women, and their vitamin D intake does not prevent it. Eur J Clin Nutr 2001; 55:1091-7.

[44]   Rucker D, Allan JA, Fick GH, Hanley DA. Vitamin D insufficiency in a population of healthy western Canadians. CMAJ 2002; 166:1517-24.

[45]   Nesby-O'Dell S, Scanlon KS, Cogswell ME *et al.* Hypovitaminosis D prevalence and determinants among African American and white women of reproductive age: third National Health and Nutrition Examination Survey, 1988-1994. Am J Clin Nutr 2002; 76:187-92.

[46]   Looker AC, Dawson-Hughes B, Calvo MS, *et al.* Serum 25-hydroxyvitamin D status of adolescents and adults in two seasonal subpopulations from NHANES III. Bone 2002; 30:771-7.

[47]   Isaia G, Giorgino R, Rini GB, *et al.* Prevalence of hypovitaminosis D in elderly women in Italy: clinical consequences and risk factors. Osteoporos Int 2003; 14:577-82.

[48]   Gessner BD, Plotnik J, Muth PT. 25-hydroxyvitamin D levels among healthy children in Alaska. J Pediatr 2003; 143:434-7.

[49]   Rockell JE, Green TJ, Skeaff CM *et al.* Season and ethnicity are determinants of serum 25-hydroxyvitamin D concentrations in New Zealand children aged 5-14 y. J Nutr 2005; 135:2602-8.

[50]   Hirani V, Primatesta P. Vitamin D concentrations among people aged 65 years and over living in private households and institutions in England: population survey. Age Ageing 2005; 34:485-91.

[51]   Holick MF, Siris ES, Binkley N *et al.* Prevalence of Vitamin D inadequacy among postmenopausal North American women receiving osteoporosis therapy. J Clin Endocrinol Metab 2005; 90:3215-24.

[52]   Zadshir A, Tareen N, Pan D, *et al.* The prevalence of hypovitaminosis D among US adults: data from the NHANES III. Ethn Dis 2005; 15:S5-101.

[53]   Wolf M, Shah A, Gutierrez O *et al.* Vitamin D levels and early mortality among incident hemodialysis patients. Kidney Int 2007; 72:1004-13.

[54]   Ginde AA, Liu MC, Camargo CA, Jr. Demographic differences and trends of vitamin D insufficiency in the US population, 1988-2004. Arch Intern Med 2009; 169:626-32.

[55]   Brot C, Vestergaard P, Kolthoff N, *et al.* Vitamin D status and its adequacy in healthy Danish perimenopausal women: relationships to dietary intake, sun exposure and serum parathyroid hormone. Br J Nutr 2001; 86 Suppl 1:S97-103.

[56]   Jacob AI, Sallman A, Santiz Z, Hollis BW. Defective photoproduction of cholecalciferol in normal and uremic humans. J Nutr 1984; 114:1313-9.

[57]   Levin A, Bakris GL, Molitch M *et al.* Prevalence of abnormal serum vitamin D, PTH, calcium, and phosphorus in patients with chronic kidney disease: results of the study to evaluate early kidney disease. Kidney Int 2007; 71:31-8.

[58]   Lips P, Wiersinga A, van Ginkel FC *et al.* The effect of vitamin D supplementation on vitamin D status and parathyroid function in elderly subjects. J Clin Endocrinol Metab 1988; 67:644-50.

[59]   Holick MF. Vitamin D deficiency. N Engl J Med 2007; 357:266-81.

[60]   DeLuca HF. Overview of general physiologic features and functions of vitamin D. Am J Clin Nutr 2004; 80:1689S-96S.

[61]   Lin R, White JH. The pleiotropic actions of vitamin D. Bioessays 2004; 26:21-8.

[62]   Dobnig H, Pilz S, Scharnagl H *et al.* Independent association of low serum 25-hydroxyvitamin d and 1,25-dihydroxyvitamin d levels with all-cause and cardiovascular mortality. Arch Intern Med 2008; 168:1340-9.

[63]   Ng K, Meyerhardt JA, Wu K *et al.* Circulating 25-hydroxyvitamin d levels and survival in patients with colorectal cancer. J Clin Oncol 2008; 26:2984-91.

[64]   Zhou W, Heist RS, Liu G *et al.* Circulating 25-hydroxyvitamin D levels predict survival in early-stage non-small-cell lung cancer patients. J Clin Oncol 2007; 25:479-85.

[65]   Heist RS, Zhou W, Wang Z *et al.* Circulating 25-hydroxyvitamin D, VDR polymorphisms, and survival in advanced non-small-cell lung cancer. J Clin Oncol 2008; 26:5596-602.

[66]   Ravani P, Malberti F, Tripepi G *et al.* Vitamin D levels and patient outcome in chronic kidney disease. Kidney Int 2009; 75:88-95.

[67]   Mehrotra R, Kermah DA, Salusky IB *et al.* Chronic kidney disease, hypovitaminosis D, and mortality in the United States. Kidney Int 2009; 76:977-83.

[68]   Kovesdy CP, Ahmadzadeh S, Anderson JE, Kalantar-Zadeh K. Association of activated vitamin D treatment and mortality in chronic kidney disease. Arch Intern Med 2008; 168:397-403.

[69]   Shoji T, Shinohara K, Kimoto E *et al.* Lower risk for cardiovascular mortality in oral 1alpha-hydroxy vitamin D3 users in a haemodialysis population. Nephrol Dial Transplant 2004; 19:179-84.

[70]   Teng M, Wolf M, Ofsthun MN *et al.* Activated injectable vitamin D and hemodialysis survival: a historical cohort study. J Am Soc Nephrol 2005; 16:1115-25.

[71]   Tentori F, Hunt WC, Stidley CA *et al*. Mortality risk among hemodialysis patients receiving different vitamin D analogs. Kidney Int 2006; 70:1858-65.

[72]   Kalantar-Zadeh K, Kuwae N, Regidor DL *et al*. Survival predictability of time-varying indicators of bone disease in maintenance hemodialysis patients. Kidney Int 2006; 70:771-80.

[73]   Melamed ML, Michos ED, Post W, Astor B. 25-hydroxyvitamin D levels and the risk of mortality in the general population. Arch Intern Med 2008; 168:1629-37.

[74]   Autier P, Gandini S. Vitamin D supplementation and total mortality: a meta-analysis of randomized controlled trials. Arch Intern Med 2007; 167:1730-7.

[75]   Kovesdy CP, Kalantar-Zadeh K. Vitamin D receptor activation and survival in chronic kidney disease. Kidney Int 2008; 73:1355-63.

[76]   Intersalt: an international study of electrolyte excretion and blood pressure. Results for 24 hour urinary sodium and potassium excretion. Intersalt Cooperative Research Group. BMJ 1988; 297:319-28.

[77]   Woodhouse PR, Khaw KT, Plummer M. Seasonal variation of blood pressure and its relationship to ambient temperature in an elderly population. J Hypertens 1993; 11:1267-74.

[78]   Cooper R, Rotimi C. Hypertension in populations of West African origin: is there a genetic predisposition? J Hypertens 1994; 12:215-27.

[79]   Rostand SG. Ultraviolet light may contribute to geographic and racial blood pressure differences. Hypertension 1997; 30:150-6.

[80]   Kunes J, Tremblay J, Bellavance F, Hamet P. Influence of environmental temperature on the blood pressure of hypertensive patients in Montreal. Am J Hypertens 1991; 4:422-6.

[81]   Krause R, Buhring M, Hopfenmuller W, *et al*. Ultraviolet B and blood pressure. Lancet 1998; 352:709-10.

[82]   Sowers MR, Wallace RB, Lemke JH. The association of intakes of vitamin D and calcium with blood pressure among women. Am J Clin Nutr 1985; 42:135-42.

[83]   Jorde R, Bonaa KH. Calcium from dairy products, vitamin D intake, and blood pressure: the Tromso Study. Am J Clin Nutr 2000; 71:1530-5.

[84]   Forman JP, Bischoff-Ferrari HA, Willett WC, *et al*. Vitamin D intake and risk of incident hypertension: results from three large prospective cohort studies. Hypertension 2005; 46:676-82.

[85]   Jacques PF, Sulsky SI, Sadowski JA, *et al*. Comparison of micronutrient intake measured by a dietary questionnaire and biochemical indicators of micronutrient status. Am J Clin Nutr 1993; 57:182-9.

[86]   Forman JP, Giovannucci E, Holmes MD *et al*. Plasma 25-hydroxyvitamin D levels and risk of incident hypertension. Hypertension 2007; 49:1063-9.

[87]   Snijder MB, Lips P, Seidell JC *et al*. Vitamin D status and parathyroid hormone levels in relation to blood pressure: a population-based study in older men and women. J Intern Med 2007; 261:558-65.

[88]   Boucher BJ, Mannan N, Noonan K, *et al*. Glucose intolerance and impairment of insulin secretion in relation to vitamin D deficiency in east London Asians. Diabetologia 1995; 38:1239-45.

[89]   Baynes KC, Boucher BJ, Feskens EJ, Kromhout D. Vitamin D, glucose tolerance and insulinaemia in elderly men. Diabetologia 1997; 40:344-7.

[90]   Scragg R, Holdaway I, Singh V, *et al*. Serum 25-hydroxyvitamin D3 levels decreased in impaired glucose tolerance and diabetes mellitus. Diabetes Res Clin Pract 1995; 27:181-8.

[91]   Scragg R, Sowers M, Bell C. Serum 25-hydroxyvitamin D, diabetes, and ethnicity in the Third National Health and Nutrition Examination Survey. Diabetes Care 2004; 27:2813-8.

[92]   Chiu KC, Chu A, Go VL, Saad MF. Hypovitaminosis D is associated with insulin resistance and beta cell dysfunction. Am J Clin Nutr 2004; 79:820-5.

[93]   Norman AW, Frankel JB, Heldt AM, Grodsky GM. Vitamin D deficiency inhibits pancreatic secretion of insulin. Science 1980; 209:823-5.

[94]   Martins D, Wolf M, Pan D *et al*. Prevalence of cardiovascular risk factors and the serum levels of 25-hydroxyvitamin D in the United States: data from the Third National Health and Nutrition Examination Survey. Arch Intern Med 2007; 167:1159-65.

[95]   Ford ES, Ajani UA, McGuire LC, Liu S. Concentrations of serum vitamin D and the metabolic syndrome among U.S. adults. Diabetes Care 2005; 28:1228-30.

[96]   Reis JP, von MD, Miller ER, III. Relation of 25-hydroxyvitamin D and parathyroid hormone levels with metabolic syndrome among US adults. Eur J Endocrinol 2008; 159:41-8.

[97]   Pilz S, Marz W, Wellnitz B *et al*. Association of vitamin D deficiency with heart failure and sudden cardiac death in a large cross-sectional study of patients referred for coronary angiography. J Clin Endocrinol Metab 2008; 93:3927-35.

[98]   Pilz S, Dobnig H, Fischer JE *et al.* Low vitamin d levels predict stroke in patients referred to coronary angiography. Stroke 2008; 39:2611-3.

[99]   Wang AY, Lam CW, Sanderson JE *et al.* Serum 25-hydroxyvitamin D status and cardiovascular outcomes in chronic peritoneal dialysis patients: a 3-y prospective cohort study. Am J Clin Nutr 2008; 87:1631-8.

[100]   Lund B, Badskjaer J, Lund B, Soerensen OH. Vitamin D and ischaemic heart disease. Horm Metab Res 1978; 10:553-6.

[101]   Scragg R, Jackson R, Holdaway IM, Lim T, Beaglehole R. Myocardial infarction is inversely associated with plasma 25-hydroxyvitamin D3 levels: a community-based study. Int J Epidemiol 1990; 19:559-63.

[102]   Fahrleitner-Pammer A, Obernosterer A, Pilger E *et al.* Hypovitaminosis D, impaired bone turnover and low bone mass are common in patients with peripheral arterial disease. Osteoporos Int 2005; 16:319-24.

[103]   Fahrleitner A, Dobnig H, Obernosterer A *et al.* Vitamin D deficiency and secondary hyperparathyroidism are common complications in patients with peripheral arterial disease. J Gen Intern Med 2002; 17:663-9.

[104]   Targher G, Bertolini L, Padovani R *et al.* Serum 25-hydroxyvitamin D3 concentrations and carotid artery intima-media thickness among type 2 diabetic patients. Clin Endocrinol (Oxf) 2006; 65:593-7.

[105]   Chonchol M, Cigolini M, Targher G. Association between 25-hydroxyvitamin D deficiency and cardiovascular disease in type 2 diabetic patients with mild kidney dysfunction. Nephrol Dial Transplant 2008; 23:269-74.

[106]   Wilke RA, Simpson RU, Mukesh BN *et al.* Genetic variation in CYP27B1 is associated with congestive heart failure in patients with hypertension. Pharmacogenomics 2009; 10:1789-97.

[107]   Kendrick J, Targher G, Smits G, Chonchol M. 25-Hydroxyvitamin D deficiency is independently associated with cardiovascular disease in the Third National Health and Nutrition Examination Survey. Atherosclerosis 2009; 205:255-60.

[108]   Melamed ML, Muntner P, Michos ED *et al.* Serum 25-hydroxyvitamin D levels and the prevalence of peripheral arterial disease: results from NHANES 2001 to 2004. Arterioscler Thromb Vasc Biol 2008; 28:1179-85.

[109]   de Boer IH, Kestenbaum B, Shoben AB, *et al.* 25-hydroxyvitamin D levels inversely associate with risk for developing coronary artery calcification. J Am Soc Nephrol 2009; 20:1805-12.

[110]   Giovannucci E, Liu Y, Hollis BW, Rimm EB. 25-hydroxyvitamin D and risk of myocardial infarction in men: a prospective study. Arch Intern Med 2008; 168:1174-80.

[111]   Wang TJ, Pencina MJ, Booth SL *et al.* Vitamin D deficiency and risk of cardiovascular disease. Circulation 2008; 117:503-11.

[112]   Ingraham BA, Bragdon B, Nohe A. Molecular basis of the potential of vitamin D to prevent cancer. Curr Med Res Opin 2008; 24:139-49.

[113]   Peterlik M, Cross HS. Dysfunction of the vitamin D endocrine system as common cause for multiple malignant and other chronic diseases. Anticancer Res 2006; 26:2581-8.

[114]   Apperly FL. The relation of solar radiation to cancer mortality in North America. Cancer Res 1941; 1:191-5.

[115]   Garland CF, Garland FC. Do sunlight and vitamin D reduce the likelihood of colon cancer? Int J Epidemiol 1980; 9:227-31.

[116]   Garland FC, Garland CF, Gorham ED, Young JF. Geographic variation in breast cancer mortality in the United States: a hypothesis involving exposure to solar radiation. Prev Med 1990; 19:614-22.

[117]   Gorham ED, Garland FC, Garland CF. Sunlight and breast cancer incidence in the USSR. Int J Epidemiol 1990; 19:820-4.

[118]   Hanchette CL, Schwartz GG. Geographic patterns of prostate cancer mortality. Evidence for a protective effect of ultraviolet radiation. Cancer 1992; 70:2861-9.

[119]   Lefkowitz ES, Garland CF. Sunlight, vitamin D, and ovarian cancer mortality rates in US women. Int J Epidemiol 1994; 23:1133-6.

[120]   Grant WB, Mohr SB. Ecological studies of ultraviolet B, vitamin D and cancer since 2000. Ann Epidemiol 2009; 19:446-54.

[121]   Giovannucci E, Liu Y, Rimm EB *et al.* Prospective study of predictors of vitamin D status and cancer incidence and mortality in men. J Natl Cancer Inst 2006; 98:451-9.

[122]   Pilz S, Dobnig H, Winklhofer-Roob B *et al.* Low serum levels of 25-hydroxyvitamin D predict fatal cancer in patients referred to coronary angiography. Cancer Epidemiol Biomarkers Prev 2008; 17:1228-33.

[123]   Freedman DM, Looker AC, Chang SC, Graubard BI. Prospective study of serum vitamin D and cancer mortality in the United States. J Natl Cancer Inst 2007; 99:1594-602.

[124]   Garland CF, Comstock GW, Garland FC, *et al.* Serum 25-hydroxyvitamin D and colon cancer: eight-year prospective study. Lancet 1989; 2:1176-8.

[125] Skinner HG, Michaud DS, Giovannucci E, *et al.* Vitamin D intake and the risk for pancreatic cancer in two cohort studies. Cancer Epidemiol Biomarkers Prev 2006; 15:1688-95.

[126] Stolzenberg-Solomon RZ, Vieth R, Azad A *et al.* A prospective nested case-control study of vitamin D status and pancreatic cancer risk in male smokers. Cancer Res 2006; 66:10213-9.

[127] Stolzenberg-Solomon RZ, Hayes RB, Horst RL, *et al.* Serum vitamin D and risk of pancreatic cancer in the prostate, lung, colorectal, and ovarian screening trial. Cancer Res 2009; 69:1439-47.

[128] Ahonen MH, Tenkanen L, Teppo L, *et al.* Prostate cancer risk and prediagnostic serum 25-hydroxyvitamin D levels (Finland). Cancer Causes Control 2000; 11:847-52.

[129] Tuohimaa P, Tenkanen L, Ahonen M *et al.* Both high and low levels of blood vitamin D are associated with a higher prostate cancer risk: a longitudinal, nested case-control study in the Nordic countries. Int J Cancer 2004; 108:104-8.

[130] Corder EH, Guess HA, Hulka BS *et al.* Vitamin D and prostate cancer: a prediagnostic study with stored sera. Cancer Epidemiol Biomarkers Prev 1993; 2:467-72.

[131] Braun MM, Helzlsouer KJ, Hollis BW, Comstock GW. Prostate cancer and prediagnostic levels of serum vitamin D metabolites (Maryland, United States). Cancer Causes Control 1995; 6:235-9.

[132] Gann PH, Ma J, Hennekens CH, Hollis BW, *et al.* Circulating vitamin D metabolites in relation to subsequent development of prostate cancer. Cancer Epidemiol Biomarkers Prev 1996; 5:121-6.

[133] Nomura AM, Stemmermann GN, Lee J *et al.* Serum vitamin D metabolite levels and the subsequent development of prostate cancer (Hawaii, United States). Cancer Causes Control 1998; 9:425-32.

[134] Jacobs ET, Giuliano AR, Martinez ME, *et al.* Plasma levels of 25-hydroxyvitamin D, 1,25-dihydroxyvitamin D and the risk of prostate cancer. J Steroid Biochem Mol Biol 2004; 89-90:533-7.

[135] Platz EA, Leitzmann MF, Hollis BW, *et al.* Plasma 1,25-dihydroxy- and 25-hydroxyvitamin D and subsequent risk of prostate cancer. Cancer Causes Control 2004; 15:255-65.

[136] Ahn J, Peters U, Albanes D *et al.* Serum vitamin D concentration and prostate cancer risk: a nested case-control study. J Natl Cancer Inst 2008; 100:796-804.

[137] Li H, Stampfer MJ, Hollis JB *et al.* A prospective study of plasma vitamin D metabolites, vitamin D receptor polymorphisms, and prostate cancer. PLoS Med 2007; 4:e103.

[138] Ingles SA, Ross RK, Yu MC *et al.* Association of prostate cancer risk with genetic polymorphisms in vitamin D receptor and androgen receptor. J Natl Cancer Inst 1997; 89:166-70.

[139] Ma J, Stampfer MJ, Gann PH *et al.* Vitamin D receptor polymorphisms, circulating vitamin D metabolites, and risk of prostate cancer in United States physicians. Cancer Epidemiol Biomarkers Prev 1998; 7:385-90.

[140] Xu Y, Shibata A, McNeal JE, *et al.* Vitamin D receptor start codon polymorphism (FokI) and prostate cancer progression. Cancer Epidemiol Biomarkers Prev 2003; 12:23-7.

[141] Chen WY, Bertone-Johnson ER, Hunter DJ, *et al.* Associations between polymorphisms in the vitamin D receptor and breast cancer risk. Cancer Epidemiol Biomarkers Prev 2005; 14:2335-9.

[142] Mucci LA, Spiegelman D. Vitamin D and prostate cancer risk--a less sunny outlook? J Natl Cancer Inst 2008; 100:759-61.

[143] Feldman D, Zhao XY, Krishnan AV. Vitamin D and prostate cancer. Endocrinology 2000; 141:5-9.

[144] Giovannucci E. Vitamin D and cancer incidence in the Harvard cohorts. Ann Epidemiol 2009; 19:84-8.

[145] Wactawski-Wende J, Kotchen JM, Anderson GL *et al.* Calcium plus vitamin D supplementation and the risk of colorectal cancer. N Engl J Med 2006; 354:684-96.

CHAPTER 4

Does Vitamin D Supplementation Improve Health?

Alan H. Lau* and Yee Ming Lee*

College of Pharmacy, University of Illinois at Chicago, Chicago, Illinois, USA

Abstract: There has been a recent plethora of studies uncovering the newly discovered physiological and pharmacological effects of vitamin D. With an increasing recognition of hypovitaminosis D worldwide, there is much interest to address the clinical significance of vitamin D deficiency and identify the most optimal regimen to replenish the body stores through supplementation. With our growing understanding of the non-mineral/bone activities of vitamin D, such as its effects on immune system, cancer and cardiovascular disease, there is a need to establish the optimal means of assessing vitamin D sufficiency and deficiency, the amount of vitamin D needed for optimal body function and how much vitamin D supplementation is required among individuals. As vitamin D is a pre-hormone that can both be synthesized in the body and obtained from the diet, there are challenges in deriving a recommendation. In addition, the amount of vitamin D present in the body is also influenced by factors such as aging, skin pigmentation, concomitant interacting medications and renal disease. For now, 25(OH)D is commonly used to determine vitamin D body stores in studies and clinical practice. This chapter seeks to discuss the issues surrounding vitamin D supplementation in the light of these new findings and address the concern over the vitamin D deficiency with the view that "more vitamin D is not necessarily better".

Keywords: Adequate intake (AI), autoimmune diseases, bone health, cancer, estimated average requirement (EAR), 25(OH)D recommendations, 25(OH)D as a biomarker, recommended dietary allowance (RDA), tolerable upper intake level (UL), U.S. Institute of Medicine (IOM), vitamin D toxicity.

INTRODUCTION

The importance of vitamin D for the development and maintenance of bone and skeletal function has been well recognized for decades. However, the recent surge in the publication of information on vitamin D beyond its conventional effects on bone health shows a growing appreciation of its broad impact on many physiological processes. As eluded in other chapters, vitamin D deficiency is a growing problem as evident in the low 25-hydroxyvitamin D (25(OH)D) levels reported among individuals in many countries. This increasing prevalence of vitamin D deficiency together with the new findings on its effects beyond bone and skeletal function compel us to examine if the current vitamin D supplementation guidelines are adequate.

In order to define the optimal vitamin D intake, we need to first understand the physiological effects of vitamin D. We would then need to identify the optimal concentration of 25(OH)D needed to achieve these actions. After which, we would examine the relationship between vitamin D intake and circulating 25(OH)D levels before finally considering the level of vitamin D intake and its adverse effects.

THE PHYSIOLOGICAL EFFECTS OF VITAMIN D

Vitamin D Production and Metabolism

Humans obtain their vitamin D from sun exposure, diet and vitamin D supplements [1, 2]. Vitamin D is available orally in two forms: vitamin D_2 (ergocalciferol) and D_3 (cholecalciferol). Both vitamin D_2 and D_3 need to undergo similar activation processes in the liver and kidney to yield the final active product, $1,25(OH)_2D$ (calcitriol).

In this chapter, vitamin D is used to represent both D_2 and D_3. The different nomenclatures of the vitamin D precursors and their metabolites are shown in Table **1**.

---

*Address correspondence to Alan H. Lau and Yee Ming Lee: College of Pharmacy, University of Illinois at Chicago, Chicago, IL, 60612, USA; E-mails: alanlau@uic.edu; ylee227@uic.edu

J. Ruth Wu-Wong (Ed)

Table 1: Nomenclature of vitamin D precursors and metabolites (adapted from [3])

Common Name	Clinical Name	Comments
Cholecalciferol	Vitamin D_3	Photosynthesized in the skin or obtained from the diet
Ergocalciferol	Vitamin D_2	Obtained from diet
Calcidiol	25(OH)D	Circulating form of vitamin D
Calcitriol	1,25(OH)$_2$D	Active form of vitamin D

As mentioned in other chapters, vitamin D_2 is found in yeast and plant ergosterol products, while vitamin D_3 is obtained from animal food products (such as fatty fish) and cutaneous photosynthesis from 7-dehydrocholesterol as shown in Fig. 1. In the human skin, 7-dehydrocholesterol absorbs ultraviolet B (UVB) radiation and is converted to pre-vitamin D_3, followed by thermal isomerization to form vitamin D_3 which is then transported in the blood *via* vitamin D-binding protein (DBP). Some of this pre-vitamin D_3 is also broken down by UVB to inactive metabolites such as tachysterol and lumisterol, limiting the cutaneous production of vitamin D_3. Therefore, excessive sun exposure cannot lead to vitamin D toxicity [4, 5]. Following the ingestion of vitamin D_2 and D_3 *via* foods or supplements, this fat-soluble vitamin is incorporated into chylomicrons within the enterocyte and reaches the systemic circulation *via* the lymphatic system. The chylomicrons are metabolized to remnant particles which then transport vitamin D to the liver.

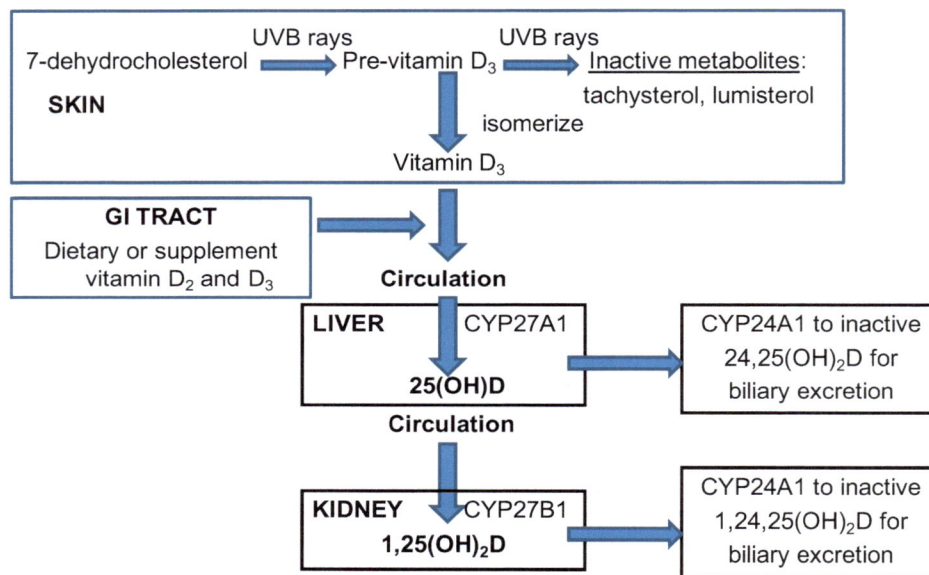

Figure 1: The process of vitamin D formation and metabolism. In the skin, 7-dehydrocholesterol is converted by UVB rays to pre-vitamin D_3 that isomerizes to vitamin D_3. Further UVB exposure converts pre-vitamin D_3 to inactive metabolites, tachysterol and lumisterol. Dietary and supplement vitamin D_2 and D_3 as well as the skin-photosynthesized vitamin D_3 are transported to the liver where CYP27A1 converts it to 25(OH)D. This inactive 25(OH)D precursor is then transported to kidney for further activation by CYP27B1 to 1,25(OH)$_2$D (calcitriol). Both 25(OH)D and 1,25(OH)$_2$D are destroyed by a ubiquitous enzyme CYP24A1 to inactive water-soluble metabolites for biliary excretion (adapted from Wolpowitz *et al.* [3]).

Vitamin D produced from cutaneous synthesis or ingested from the diet does not circulate in the blood for long as it is readily taken up by adipose tissue or liver for storage or activation. In the liver, both vitamin D_2 and D_3 are hydroxylated by the cytochrome P450 enzyme 25-hydroxylase (CYP27A1) to 25(OH)D. This inactive precursor, 25(OH)D, is the major circulating form of vitamin D in human. 25(OH)D is then activated in the kidney *via* 25-hydroxyvitamin D_3 1-alpha-hydroxylase (CYP27B1, 1α-hydroxylase) to the biologically active form of vitamin D, 1,25(OH)$_2$D (calcitriol). Both 25(OH)D and 1,25(OH)$_2$D are broken down by an ubiquitous enzyme CYP24A1 (1,25-dihydroxyvitamin D_3 24-hydroxylase or 24-hydroxylase) to inactive products such as calcitroic acid that are biliary excreted.

The renal production of 1,25(OH)$_2$D (calcitriol) is tightly regulated by various factors including two counteracting hormones, parathyroid hormone (PTH) and fibroblast growth factor 23 (FGF-23) in response to serum calcium and phosphorus levels [6]. Low serum calcium or phosphate levels stimulate PTH production that in turn up-regulates 1,25(OH)$_2$D synthesis, while high phosphate levels stimulate FGF-23 release resulting in phosphaturia and inhibition of 1,25(OH)$_2$D synthesis [7]. In the plasma, the activated vitamin D metabolite, 1,25(OH)$_2$D is transported by the vitamin D-binding protein (DBP) to its target organs where it binds to a nuclear receptor, the vitamin D receptor (VDR) [1, 8, 9]. Activated VDR then interacts with numerous co-factors to form a transcriptional complex that binds to specific DNA sequences known as vitamin D response elements that regulate gene transcription.

The Classical and Non-Classical Physiological Effects of Vitamin D

The classical effect of vitamin D on calcium and phosphate homeostasis is mediated by VDR's effects on the intestine, bone, parathyroid and kidney after the receptor is activated by 1,25(OH)$_2$D [1]. When serum calcium is low, calcium-sensing proteins in the parathyroid gland detect this, and PTH is released to stimulate CYP27B1 and increase 1,25(OH)$_2$D production. 1,25(OH)$_2$D binds to and activates VDR, leading to up-regulation of genes involved in increasing calcium and phosphorus absorption in the intestine. It also works with PTH to stimulate the production of the Receptor Activator Nuclear Factor–κB ligand (RANKL) by osteoclasts, resulting in osteoclastogenesis and calcium-phosphate mobilization from the bone. PTH also works with 1,25(OH)$_2$D to stimulate renal distal tubular calcium reabsorption to restore serum calcium levels. As calcium levels normalize, PTH secretion is suppressed.

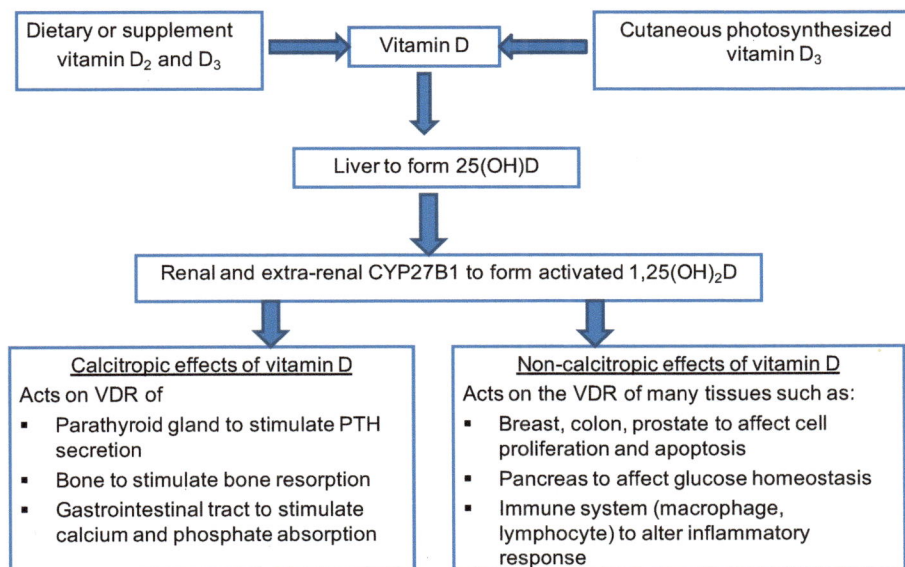

Figure 2: The calcitriopic and non-calcitropic effects of 1,25(OH)$_2$D formed in renal and extra-renal tissues (adapted from Maalouf [10]).

The discovery that tissues outside the kidney (such as the colon and prostate) express the CYP27B1 enzyme to convert circulating 25(OH)D to 1,25(OH)$_2$D, as well as the presence of VDR in tissues not involved with the calcitropic effects of vitamin D, implies that vitamin D exerts other non-classical (non-calcitropic) effects beyond calcium and phosphate homeostasis [4, 8, 10-13]. Vitamin D response elements are present in a large number of genes involved in a variety of non-classical roles such as regulating cancer cell growth, renin production and modifying immunomodulatory effects of T and B lymphocytes. Therefore, in addition to the endocrine effects of 1,25(OH)$_2$D produced from the kidney, locally produced 1,25(OH)$_2$D in extra-renal tissues could act in an autocrine and/or paracrine manner to exert the non-calcitropic effects of vitamin D as shown in Fig. **2**. This has led to the concept that adequate 25(OH)D levels may be required for vitamin D regulation of a large number of physiological functions beyond that of the classical bone mineral effect.

THE CONCENTRATION OF VITAMIN D TO ACHIEVE ITS PHYSIOLOGICAL EFFECTS

The Use of 25(OH)D as A Biomarker

Serum 25(OH)D is widely used as a marker of vitamin D nutriture. It is currently regarded as the best indicator of the net contribution of vitamin D from cutaneous synthesis, dietary intake and vitamin D supplementation [14]. Serum 25(OH)D level may therefore reflect the body's vitamin D stores and hence be used as a "biomarker of exposure" to determine the intake of vitamin D. However, it is unclear to what extent does this 25(OH)D level serve as a "biomarker of effect", whereby how does the 25(OH)D level correlate with health outcomes causally or does it serve as a predictor of health outcomes instead.

It is important to note that although the physiological effects of vitamin D are mediated by the activated form of vitamin D, $1,25(OH)_2D$, the levels of $1,25(OH)_2D$ have not been used typically to measure vitamin D nutriture or as a marker of vitamin D health outcomes in studies [3]. 25(OH)D is used instead of $1,25(OH)_2D$, as $1,25(OH)_2D$ has a short half-life of 10 to 20 hours compared to the longer half-life of 15 days with 25(OH)D [15]. In addition, $1,25(OH)_2D$ level can be normal or elevated in the presence of vitamin D deficiency, due to the body's response by upregulating CYP27B1 to convert circulating 25(OH)D to $1,25(OH)_2D$, as well as the effect of secondary hyperparathyroidism [6].

Current 25(OH)D Recommendations Based On Bone Health Outcomes

The U.S. Institute of Medicine (IOM) had published in 1997 a report on Dietary Reference Intakes (DRI) for various nutrients such as calcium and vitamin D [16]. For vitamin D, bone health was the basis for deriving DRI with 25(OH)D level as an indicator of bone health outcomes. DRIs are reference values used in planning and assessing diets for healthy populations by the National Academy of Sciences. They encompass the Estimated Average Requirement (EAR), the Recommended Dietary Allowance (RDA), the Adequate Intake (AI), and the Tolerable Upper Intake Level (UL) which are defined in Table **2**. It is important to note that DRIs are developed for "normal healthy persons" in the North American population and not for individuals with different disease states.

Table 2: Definition of the different terms used in dietary reference recommendations [16]

Term	Definition
Estimated Average Requirement (EAR)	The nutrient intake value to meet the requirement defined by a specified indicator of adequacy in 50% of the individuals in a life stage.
Recommended Dietary Allowance (RDA)	The average daily dietary intake level sufficient to meet the nutrient requirements of at least 97.5% of the population.
Adequate Intake (AI)	This is used instead of an RDA, when there is insufficient scientific evidence to calculate an EAR. It is based on observed or experimentally determined estimates of the average nutrient intake by a group of healthy people.
Tolerable Upper Intake Level (UL)	This is the highest level of daily nutrient intake that will pose no risks of adverse health effects to almost all individuals in the general population. As intake increases above the UL, the risk of adverse effects increases.

For vitamin D, the 1997 IOM report concluded that there was insufficient data to provide EAR and RDA due to the uncertainties about cutaneous exposure, dietary vitamin D content and vitamin D stores, so AI was used (Table **3**). The AI of vitamin D was based on the amount needed to maintain a defined criterion of adequacy (*e.g.* prevent rickets or osteomalacia) in a healthy population. Since then, more studies on vitamin D were published that allowed a separation of the contribution from sun exposure and dietary vitamin D intake to be estimated and the IOM 2011 report is now able to provide the DRI of calcium and vitamin D for bone health (Table **3**).

Despite the new data after the 1997 IOM report, the 2011 IOM reporting committee acknowledged the lack of intervention trials looking at the dose-response relationships of nutrients [14]. Most data were derived from a single dose vitamin D that was often relatively high; with many studies often using calcium and vitamin D combinations, making it difficult to discern the effects of each nutrient alone. The DRIs of vitamin D in the 2011 IOM report was based on the assumption of minimal or no sun exposure. In addition, with the effects of calcium and vitamin D being so intertwined, the DRIs for one nutrient rests on the premise that the intake of other nutrient was being met.

Table 3: 1997 and 2011 IOM recommendations on the dietary reference intake of vitamin D for the different life stage groups with minimal sun exposure [14, 16]

Life Stage Group	1997 Recommendations		2011 Recommendations		
	Adequate intake (AI) (IU/day)	Upper level intake (UL) (IU/day)	Estimated average requirement (IU/day)	Recommended dietary allowance (IU/day)	Upper level of intake/ day (IU/day)
Infants 0 to 6 months	200	1000	**	**	1000
Infants 6 to 12 months			**	**	1500
1 to 3 years old		2000	400	600	2500
4 to 8 years old					3000
9 to 50 years old					4000
51 to 70 years old	400				
>70 years old	600			800	
14 to 50 years old pregnant/lactating	200			600	

** For infants, adequate intake is 400 IU/day for 0 to 12 months.

25(OH) Level as A Biomarker of Vitamin D Status

Definition of Vitamin D Sufficiency

Currently, there is no consensus on the definition of vitamin D deficiency. What is commonly used is the level of 25(OH)D that causes maximal PTH suppression, since PTH promotes bone loss [17]. Severely low 25(OH)D <10 ng/mL has been associated with cortical bone loss and increased fractures. Some have defined vitamin D deficiency as 25(OH)D levels <20 ng/mL and sufficiency as >30 ng/mL. The utility of correlating serum 25(OH)D concentration to PTH suppression needs to take into account that PTH is affected by other factors such as age, gender, weight and calcium intake. Many studies have reported serum 25(OH)D causing PTH suppression at a range of 10 to 50 ng/mL and one recent review has proposed the definition of vitamin D insufficiency as serum 25(OH)D <20 ng/mL [18]. One needs to take this into consideration that different studies use slightly different serum 25(OH)D cut-offs in their definition of vitamin D deficiency. The 2011 IOM report has defined vitamin D status as shown in Table **4**. Based on this 2011 IOM definition, the Centers for Disease Control and Prevention health statistics report on the vitamin D status of the US population for 2001 to 2006 found that 67% of the population had sufficient 25(OH)D while 24% were at risk of inadequacy and 8% were at risk of deficiency [19]. Overall, the risk of vitamin D deficiency increased between 1988 to 1994 and 2001 to 2002 in both genders, but did not change between the periods 2001 to 2002 and 2005 to 2006.

Table 4: The 2011 IOM definition of vitamin D status based on serum 25(OH)D levels [14]

25(OH)D Levels	IOM 2010 Definition of Vitamin D Status
<12 ng/mL (30 nmol/L)	At risk of vitamin D deficiency
12 to 19 ng/mL (30-49 nmol/L)	At risk for vitamin D inadequacy
20 to 50 ng/mL (50-125 nmol/L)	Sufficient in vitamin D
>50 ng/mL (125 nmol/L)	Possibly harmful vitamin D

25(OH)D Levels, Vitamin D Supplementation on Bone Health

Serum 25(OH)D levels are commonly used to assess vitamin D status in trials evaluating bone health outcomes such as fracture and falls. In a study where adults with low serum 25(OH)D level between 11 to

19 ng/mL were given vitamin D supplementation, there was a substantial decrease in PTH concentration, whereas those with 25(OH)D level of 20 to 25 ng/mL had no substantial PTH change [20]. Vitamin D deficiency was thus defined as 25(OH)D level of <20 ng/mL. In another study in post-menopausal women with 25(OH)D level of >30 ng/mL, no increase in intestinal calcium absorption was observed. Holick therefore suggested that vitamin D sufficiency be defined as serum 25(OH)D >30 ng/mL while those with level between 21-29 ng/mL are considered having vitamin D insufficiency [17].

Although the optimal 25(OH)D level for bone health can be determined using the PTH level, bone mineral density (BMD) and fracture risk may be a better endpoint. In the elderly, BMD is a predictor of fracture risk. In a National Health and Nutrition Examination Survey (NHANES III) 1988 and 1994, higher serum 25(OH)D was associated with higher BMD and appeared to plateau in the range of 36 to 40 ng/mL in elderly white [21]. This would lead one to ask if the improvement in BMD associated with vitamin D supplementation might translate to reduction in falls and fractures.

A meta-analysis of randomized controlled trials found a dose-response relationship between vitamin D and non-vertebral fracture reduction among the elderly $\geq$ 65 years, with higher vitamin D doses 482 to 770 IU/day reducing non-vertebral fractures by at least 20% and hip fractures by at least 18%, independent of calcium supplementation [22]. Another analysis found that oral vitamin D dose of 400 IU/day was not sufficient for fracture prevention while higher doses of 700 to 800 IU/day reduced hip and non-vertebral fractures in ambulatory and institutionalized elderly [23]. The large Women's Health Initiative study that compared vitamin D 400 IU/day plus calcium 1000 mg versus placebo confirmed the findings that low dose vitamin D had no benefit in reducing hip fracture [24]. Based on the BMD results and studies on the prevention of hip and non-vertebral fractures in older adults, serum 25(OH)D of 30 to 40ng/mL seemed to be the optimal level for maintaining bone health [25, 26].

Since many bone health studies had vitamin D co-administered with calcium, will vitamin D alone confer any protective bone effect? A Cochrane meta-analysis found that vitamin D in combination with calcium reduced hip fractures (RR 0.84, 95% CI 0.73 to 0.96), but vitamin D alone was unlikely to be effective in preventing hip fractures (RR 1.15; 95% CI 0.99 to 1.33), vertebral fractures (RR 0.90; 95% CI 0.42 to 1.92) or any new fracture (RR 1.01; 95% CI 0.93 to 1.09) [25].

One key limitation in interpreting vitamin D trials on bone health is the inconsistent reporting of baseline 25(OH)D since individuals with low baseline 25(OH)D level would be expected to benefit most from vitamin D supplementation. In addition, fractures and BMD are long term bone effects which other factors such as the amount of calcium intake, tobacco smoking and exercise can have confounding influence, hence a single point measurement of 25(OH)D may not be a specific biomarker of bone health [27]. As such, 25(OH)D is not as a "biomarker of effect" but is the current available biomarker of vitamin D exposure [14].

Based on the current studies on bone health, there is a dose-response relationship between vitamin D supplementation and 25(OH)D levels, with higher oral vitamin D dose of at least 700 IU/day being required to prevent falls and fractures [23]. It is recommended to monitor and maintain adequate 25(OH)D levels of around 30 ng/mL [25, 26], with additional calcium supplementation to be considered for individuals with low dietary calcium intake.

25(OH)D Levels, Vitamin D Supplementation on Fall and Physical Performance

While the protective benefit of vitamin D on fracture has been established on the basis of its effect on calcium and phosphate homeostasis, it has been suggested that vitamin D may also improve muscle strength. This physiological effect may be mediated by the binding of the active $1,25(OH)_2D$ to VDR in the muscle tissue, leading to *de novo* protein synthesis and muscle cell growth [28]. In addition, $1,25(OH)_2D$ regulates calcium uptake by the muscle, which in turn controls muscle contraction, hence affecting the risk for falls and physical performance [14].

One meta-analysis of randomized double-blind controlled trials reported that vitamin D supplementation reduced the risk of falls in the elderly by 22% (95% CI 0.64 to 0.92) compared to calcium or placebo [28].

However, these trials used different vitamin D doses and vitamin D analogs, so no specific vitamin D dose could be recommended. The effect of vitamin D on reducing the risk of falls was not consistently seen in other studies [14]. Due to the inconsistent findings, there is currently insufficient evidence to provide any vitamin D supplementation dose for reducing the risk of falls and improving physical performance.

25(OH)D Levels, Vitamin D Supplementation and Mortality From Any Cause

An observational study of more than 13,000 adults from the NHANES III (1988 to 1994) showed that low 25(OH)D levels of <18 ng/mL was independently associated with higher risk of all-cause mortality in the general population [29]. Other epidemiological studies have also observed an increased risk of chronic diseases such as diabetes, multiple sclerosis, hypertension and death from common cancers associated with vitamin D deficient individuals living in higher latitude where sun exposure is reduced [2]. This led to the question of whether vitamin D supplementation could reduce mortality from chronic diseases.

A meta-analysis of randomized controlled trials found that vitamin D supplementation from 300 IU to 2000 IU/day was associated with a 7% reduction (95% CI 0.87 to 0.99) in mortality from any cause [30]. However, this meta-analysis was confounded by factors such as different types of patients studied in the different trials (healthy patients to patients with heart failure), varying baseline 25(OH)D levels from 8.8 to 30 ng/mL, varying compliance to vitamin D supplement intake from 47.7% to 95%, and a short duration of follow-up from 6 months to 7 years that might be insufficient to observe any survival benefits [31]. As such it is hard to conclude if vitamin D supplementation will definitely reduce mortality. While further studies are needed to derive any conclusion, it is important to be aware of the potential protective effects of vitamin D in light of the growing literature on its pleiotropic effects.

25(OH)D Levels, Vitamin D Supplementation and Cardiovascular Outcomes

Prospective cohort studies have found 25(OH)D levels to be inversely associated with increased cardiovascular disease mortality [32, 33]. In the Framing Offspring Study, 25(OH)D level <15 ng/mL was associated with an adjusted hazard ratio of 1.62 for incident cardiovascular disease compared with 25(OH)D levels >15 ng/mL [34].

The impact of deficiency in VDR activation on cardiovascular disease is clearly demonstrated in patients with end-stage renal disease (ESRD), where the damaged kidney is unable to convert circulating 25(OH)D to 1,25(OH)$_2$D. Cardiovascular diseases such as coronary artery disease, myocardial infarction are more prevalent among dialysis patients [35], with dialysis patients having 10 to 20 times higher risk of cardiovascular mortality rate than the general population [34].

Several mechanisms by which deficiency in VDR activation adversely affects cardiovascular function have been proposed. They include secondary hyperparathyroidism, increased activity of the renin-angiotensin-aldosterone-system (RAAS) and altered immune system [36]. Secondary hyperparathyroidism was thought to be a primary cause of cardiac dysfunction in ESRD patients. It is now recognized that direct activation of VDRs by 1,25(OH)$_2$D can reduce left ventricular hypertrophy and cardiovascular mortality [36]. In addition, parathyroidectomy in ESRD patients does not consistently reverse hypertension and left ventricular hypertrophy, suggesting that secondary hyperparathyroidism may not be the only cause of cardiovascular dysfunction and VDR could have direct effects on the cardiovascular system apart from regulating parathyroid hormone levels. The physiological effects of VDR on the myocardium were seen in animal studies, where VDR knockout mice had accelerated rates of cardiac contraction and relaxation compared with wild type mice [34]. VDR has been shown to be a negative regulator of RAAS, where VDR knockout mice were found to have increased renin, angiotensin II and aldosterone levels, and developed hypertension, cardiac hypertrophy and increased water intake [37]. VDR also has immunomodulatory actions that inhibit the inflammatory process involved in intimal and medial calcification [34].

Despite the postulated pathophysiology of VDR in cardiovascular disease, studies looking at the correlation between 25(OH)D levels and blood pressure in non-dialysis patients revealed conflicting results [36]. When the effect of vitamin D supplementation on blood pressure was examined in a prospective randomized controlled trial involving a small group of women using vitamin D_3 800 IU/day plus 1200 mg elemental calcium *versus* calcium alone, a significant reduction in systolic blood pressure and heart rate was noted [36]. Another smaller trial involving 34 diabetics given single doses of vitamin D_2 100,000 IU also showed a reduction in systolic blood pressure when compared to placebo. As both trials were only conducted for a short period of 2 months, it is uncertain if the vitamin D effects would be sustained to provide long-term cardiovascular benefits. A recent systematic review showed that low 25(OH)D levels correlated with increased incident hypertension and cardiovascular disease, but vitamin D supplementation had no effect on hypertension and cardiovascular outcomes [38]. One needs to note that there was substantial heterogeneity among the trials (such as variation in vitamin D doses and thresholds) which may have confounded the analysis.

The use of vitamin D analogs in dialysis patients showed more conclusive benefits, with vitamin D analog therapy reducing left ventricular hypertrophy [34-36, 39, 40]. Treatment of dialysis patients with active vitamin D compounds have been associated with enhanced survival compared with the untreated group [41]. The choice of vitamin D analogue seemed to matter, as observed in a historical cohort study on hemodialysis patients where the group who received paricalcitol showed a better survival than the group that received calcitriol (mortality rate was 0.180 *versus* 0.223 per person-year respectively, P <0.001) [42]. The therapeutic window of calcitriol is narrower compared to vitamin D analogs such as paricalcitol, with calcitriol having a higher potential to cause hypercalcemia [43]. As such, treatment with vitamin D analogs must be balanced against the risk of hypervitaminosis D, hypercalcemia and hyperphosphatemia that can induce vascular calcification thereby contributing towards cardiovascular mortality. There is evidence to suggest a U-shaped curve for vitamin D and cardiovascular outcomes, wherein low vitamin D levels are associated with cardiovascular calcification but treatment with high dose of vitamin D is also associated with vascular calcification [44].

Currently, vitamin D analogs are used in chronic kidney disease patients to manage secondary hyperparathyroidism with PTH as a marker to guide management. Future studies on vitamin D analogs in managing cardiovascular disease would need to identify suitable markers to monitor its therapeutic use. Although research has unraveled the possible mechanisms by which VDR regulates the cardiovascular system and observational studies have correlated vitamin D deficiency with adverse cardiovascular outcomes, the use of vitamin D supplement in non-CKD (chronic kidney disease) patients to reduce cardiovascular disease has been inconclusive [14]. As there is insufficient evidence to support the causal relationship between vitamin D supplementation and cardiovascular disease, further trials would be needed before any recommendation can be made.

25(OH)D Levels, Vitamin D Supplementation and Cancer

In vitro studies using human malignant cells lines have found that $1,25(OH)_2D$ can reduce cell proliferation, induce growth arrest and promote cellular differentiation [45, 46], and tumor cell proliferation is inhibited by vitamin D analogs that activate VDR directly [47]. In 1937, Peller first proposed that sun exposure may reduce cancer risk [48]. Since then, other findings have supported this proposal with epidemiological studies showing low vitamin D levels associated with increased risks for colon, breast and prostate cancer. Most of the research on vitamin D and cancer has focused on colorectal, prostate and breast cancers [48].

For breast cancer, *in vitro* cell studies show that $1,25(OH)_2D$ has anticancer effects [49]. However, observational studies failed to show any significant association between higher 25(OH)D levels and a reduction in breast cancer risk [14]. Prospective studies using 25(OH)D levels measured years before the breast cancer diagnosis also failed to observe any association [50]; the 25(OH)D levels reported were single time point measurements with a variable time period between the measurement and breast cancer diagnosis. The effect of vitamin D and calcium supplementation on breast cancer was studied in a few randomized controlled trials and no association was seen [14]. Given the paucity of randomized controlled trials, more interventional studies involving repeated 25(OH)D measurements before the diagnosis of breast cancer, and studies looking at the vitamin D exposure time prior to breast cancer will be needed before any vitamin D supplementation can be recommended.

In contrast, the correlation between vitamin D and colorectal cancer is stronger, with epidemiological studies showing low UVB exposure associated with increased risk for colorectal cancer [48]. An inverse correlation was observed between 25(OH)D levels and colorectal cancer, with a 50% lower incidence of colorectal cancer in individuals with 25(OH)D levels ≥33 ng/mL as compared with those with levels ≤12 ng/mL [51]. The large randomized double-blind controlled Women's Health Initiative study comparing calcium and vitamin D 400 IU/day supplementation versus placebo over 7 years found no effect of supplementation on the incidence of colorectal cancer [52]. The authors of the Women's Health Initiative study acknowledged that the lack of benefit could be due to several factors: compliance issue since the participants were allowed to take their own calcium and vitamin D, the low vitamin D dose used, the high non-adherence rate in the study, and the 7-year follow-up not long enough to demonstrate an effect on the incidence of colorectal cancer that has a latency of 10 to 20 years. In contrast, the study by Lappe *et al.* involving postmenopausal women randomized to either calcium and a higher vitamin D dose of 1100 IU/day *versus* calcium or placebo given over 4 years, found a lower relative risk of cancer in the calcium and vitamin D group than the placebo group [53]. The higher vitamin dose used raised the 25(OH)D levels significantly from 28 ng/mL to 38 ng/mL in 1 year, in contrast to the Women's Health Initiative study that had a lower baseline 25(OH)D level of 17 ng/mL and no subsequent 25(OH)D level reported. Given the conflicting findings, further studies are needed to define the vitamin D supplementation dose and duration for colorectal cancer before any dose recommendations can be made.

The data on prostate cancer has been inconclusive to show any association between vitamin D and the risk of prostate cancer [48]. While high calcium and milk intake seemed to help colorectal cancer, it worsened the risk of aggressive or advanced prostate cancer, suggesting that not all cancers respond to vitamin D in a similar manner [48]. It has been proposed that prostate cancer cells may have diminished CYP27B1 activity to convert circulating 25(OH)D to $1,25(OH)_2D$ locally at the cellular level, hence prostate cancer cells would depend more on circulating $1,25(OH)_2D$ to exert its effect on cell differentiation and proliferation. Further randomized controlled trials examining the effect of vitamin D on prostate cancer are needed before any vitamin D supplementation can be recommended.

Overall, there are insufficient randomized controlled interventional trials looking at vitamin D and cancer as the primary outcome, leaving gaps in the understanding of the causal relationship between vitamin D and the different cancers [14]. Further randomized controlled trials looking at the effect of vitamin D supplementation on different cancers will be needed with trials adequately controlled for confounding risk factors specific to the different cancers (such as diet).

25(OH)D Levels, Vitamin D Supplementation and the Immune Response to Infection

Interest in the potential role of vitamin D in modulating the immune response was generated by findings of VDR on T-lymphocytes and macrophages, activated macrophages having CYP27B1 to produce $1,25(OH)_2D$ locally and $1,25(OH)_2D$ being able to inhibit T-cell growth [54]. Unlike the renal production of $1,25(OH)_2D$ that is regulated by calcium levels, extra-renal production of $1,25(OH)_2D$ by the immune cells is regulated by immune inputs such as interferon-γ and stimulation of the toll-like-receptor-(TLR) pathogen-recognition receptor [54-58]. The innate immune response also involves the activation of TLR in polymorphonuclear cells, monocytes and macrophages that interact with specific membrane patterns shed by infectious agents. These activated macrophages and dendritic cells express CYP27B1 to produce $1,25(OH)_2D$ that induces the synthesis of the antibacterial proteins such as cathelicidin.

The role of vitamin D in infection was studied extensively for tuberculosis, where $1,25(OH)_2D$ was found to inhibit the growth of *M. tuberculosis* in cultured human macrophages [59]. This inhibition occurred when the cells were exposed to adequate levels of 25(OH)D, demonstrating that the downstream response after VDR activation depended on serum 25(OH)D levels. This also provides an explanation for the different susceptibility of different ethnic groups to *M. tuberculosis*, with African-Americans having a higher susceptibility to develop more severe *M. tuberculosis*. The higher incidence of 25(OH)D deficiency among the African-American population may be secondary to their higher skin melanin levels that compete with 7-dehydrocholesterol for UVB, resulting in less cutaneous vitamin D_3 production endogenously and hence lower 25(OH)D levels [1, 2]. Liu *et al.* found lower serum 25(OH)D levels were associated with reduced induction of the antibacterial protein, cathelicidin, in the African-American cohort compared with the Caucasian cohort [59].

Is there a role for vitamin D supplementation in treating infection? A meta-analysis found five prospective randomized placebo-controlled studies evaluating the effect of vitamin D supplementation on the treatment or prevention of bacteria infection: 4 trials for tuberculosis (TB) and 1 trial for *H. pylori* infection [60]. Four of the TB trials yielded mixed results. In a study by Martineau *et al.* [60], a single dose of 100,000 IU ergocalciferol was given to 131 TB patients, which resulted in the immunologic control of the blood bacilli Calmette-Guerin (a *M. tuberculosis* surrogate). In another study involving 24 children treated with 1000 IU vitamin D daily, there was a higher rate of TB symptom resolution than the placebo group. In the study by Nursyam *et al.* [60], treatment with 10,000 IU vitamin D daily in 67 adults with pulmonary TB for 6 weeks showed a higher rate of sputum conversion *versus* placebo group (P = 0.002). The largest prospective TB trial was reported by Wejse in 2009 [60]. It involved 365 patients treated with 100,000 IU vitamin D at baseline, 5 months and 8 months of the TB therapy. The 25(OH)D level of the treatment group increased over time but similar 25(OH)D increments were also observed in the placebo group, suggesting that the dose of vitamin D used in the intervention group may not be sufficient. This trial found no difference in sputum conversion between both groups. As such, the studies on vitamin D supplementation in TB have been hampered by limitations such as small sample size and lack of information if vitamin D dose was sufficient to replete vitamin D. In addition, VDR polymorphisms in humans have also been reported, which can affect the immune response to bacterial pathogens. Hence, further prospective intervention-based trials are needed before any recommendation can be made on vitamin D supplementation for the treatment of TB [60].

An interventional study on vitamin D treatment of *H. pylori* was conducted in 15 elderly who were given vitamin D 40 IU/day for 20 years *versus* placebo (19 elderly). Even though the *H. pylori* serology in the vitamin D group was lower (P <0.05), the absence of baseline and follow-up vitamin D levels precludes any conclusion whether the low dose vitamin D given was appropriate or not. As such, the role of vitamin D in treating *H. pylori* infection remains inconclusive [60].

25(OH)D Levels, Vitamin D Supplementation in Autoimmune Diseases and Chronic Diseases

Epidemiological studies have reported a latitudinal association between vitamin D deficiency and autoimmune diseases (such as multiple sclerosis, rheumatoid arthritis, type 1 diabetes) [2, 57, 61] and chronic diseases (such as type 2 diabetes) [62]. In a meta-analysis of observational studies evaluating the effect of vitamin D supplementation on type 1 diabetes, vitamin D supplementation in early childhood was found to associate with a lower risk of the disease [63]. Limitations of these studies in the meta-analysis include the lack of 25(OH)D levels to assess if the vitamin D doses given were adequate, incomplete information on the amount of vitamin D supplement, and the reliance on the retrospective recall by the mothers if they had given the vitamin D regularly [3, 63, 64]. Future randomized controlled trials with long period of follow-up are needed to confirm causality between vitamin D supplementation and prevention of type 1 diabetes, and to establish the best dose and duration of supplementation. Since $1,25(OH)_2D$ also affects other cytokines involved in conditions such as psoriasis, inflammatory bowel disease [54, 56], respiratory health [65] and septicemia [66], studies are ongoing to look at the therapeutic potential of vitamin D and its analogs for these autoimmune diseases.

The role of $1,25(OH)_2D$ having direct and indirect effects on insulin secretion and action has been supported by various *in vitro* and animal studies [67]. Observational studies suggest an association between low vitamin D and calcium intake and the risk of type 2 diabetes, but these findings were not adjusted for confounders such as obesity, which could predispose individuals to type 2 diabetes and contribute to lower 25(OH)D levels as a result of sequestration of vitamin D into adipose tissue [14]. In addition, the vitamin D and calcium levels were measured in patients with glucose intolerance or established diabetes, which might not reflect the levels prior to diagnosis. Therefore a causal relationship could not be established based on these observational studies. There are a few interventional studies using vitamin D with or without calcium supplementation with type 2 diabetes as the primary outcome. These studies were also inconclusive, as they were limited by the short study duration and small sample size [14, 67]. While the current findings suggest that vitamin D and calcium deficiency affect insulin response, the relative contribution of each nutrient to the type 2 diabetes risk has yet to be established. Further large randomized controlled trials will be needed to define the clinical role of vitamin D and calcium supplementation in the prevention and management of type 2 diabetes.

In summary, although there have been many studies that examine the non-classical role of vitamin D in cancer, cardiovascular disease, infection, autoimmune diseases, chronic diseases and overall mortality, there are insufficient data to conclusively derive any recommendation for vitamin D supplementation for these conditions.

THE RELATIONSHIP BETWEEN VITAMIN D INTAKE AND 25(OH) LEVELS

Vitamin D body store is often assessed according to the 25(OH)D level. However, it is difficult to plot a dose-response relationship between vitamin D supplement and 25(OH)D levels, since vitamin D is a pre-hormone that the body obtains from dietary sources and cutaneous synthesis after sun exposure. When dietary vitamin D intake is insufficient, the body compensates by increasing the cutaneous synthesis of vitamin D. The amount of vitamin D available to be convert to 25(OH)D is affected by many factors such as:

The Amount of Cutaneous Vitamin D Synthesized

The widespread use of sunscreens, the use of sunscreens with higher sun protection factor, cultural differences in dress and reduction in outdoor physical activity all can affect the amount of vitamin D cutaneously formed [2]. In addition, certain ethnic groups have higher skin melanin content, such as dark-skinned African-Americans, leading to decreased production of vitamin D_3 by as much as 99% [2, 6]. The amount of UVB rays and intensity that reach the earth varies with season and latitude, affecting the amount of sun exposure among individuals living in the temperate and tropical areas. In addition, the amount of 7-dehydrocholesterol present in the skin decreases with aging, with a 70-year old having approximately 25% of the content of a young adult, leading to a significant reduction in the skin photosynthesis of vitamin D_3.

Factors Affecting Dietary Absorption, Metabolism Distribution and Synthesis of Vitamin D

The presence of malabsorptive conditions (such as Crohn's disease) and the concurrent use of medications (such as orlistat) that can bind to fat-soluble vitamins reduce dietary absorption of vitamin D [6]. The CYP450 catabolism of vitamin D can be enhanced by medications such as anticonvulsants and highly active anti-retroviral drugs. The sequestration of fat-soluble vitamin D to the adipose tissue for storage also explains why obesity is associated with vitamin D deficiency [2, 6]. In addition, obese individuals tend to be inactive with reduced outdoor sun exposure time, thus reducing skin production of vitamin D_3. As vitamin D precursors require activation *via* liver and kidney hydroxylation, the presence of liver and/or renal impairment will hamper the vitamin D conversion process. Another possible cause of vitamin D deficiency in the general population is in exclusively breastfed infants of mothers who are already vitamin D deficient. The breast milk of such women will have low vitamin D content, leading their exclusively breastfed infants to become vitamin D deficient. As such the American Academy of Pediatrics recommends all infants, including those exclusively breastfed to receive a minimum of vitamin D 400 IU daily soon after birth [68].

Other Factors

Other factors that contribute toward vitamin D deficiency include acquired disorders such as hyperthyroidism (enhanced 25(OH)D metabolism) and genetic disorders such as mutation of the VDR gene [6].

As it is difficult to estimate the contribution made by sun exposure, current IOM DRIs are developed with the assumption of minimal sun exposure. In addition, current vitamin D supplementation guidelines are developed from studies that use serum 25(OH)D as a biomarker of bone health. Future studies will need to evaluate what is the appropriate level of 25(OH)D as a biomarker for the non-classical effects of vitamin D, and/or identify biomarkers that correlate with VDR activation at the molecular level.

WHICH VITAMIN D TO USE - VITAMIN D₂ OR D₃?

Vitamin D supplement is available as ergocalciferol (vitamin D_2) or cholecalciferol (vitamin D_3). In North America, vitamin D_2 (ergocalciferol) is available for prescription use while vitamin D_3 (cholecalciferol) is available over-the-counter in many multivitamins or as a separate nutrient. Since 1930s, both forms of vitamin D have been regarded as being equivalent and interchangeable. However, recent studies suggest that there may be some difference in potency between vitamin D_2 and D_3 [69, 70]. Oral administration of the same dose of vitamin D_2 and D_3 increases 25(OH)D level differently, with vitamin D_2 having a third of the potency of vitamin D_3 in terms of its ability to increase serum 25(OH)D. In addition vitamin D_2 has a shorter duration of action. The proposed mechanism of vitamin D_3 in maintaining higher 25(OH)D concentrations could be due to its greater binding affinity to vitamin D binding protein, leading to a longer circulating half-life and slower clearance from the circulation, and also due to its higher affinity for the liver CYP27A1 enzyme for its conversion to $25(OH)D_3$. However, a recent study showed no difference in vitamin D_2 and D_3 in maintaining circulating 25(OH)D [71]. Based on the findings, the 2011 IOM committee states that without further studies, a firm conclusion on the different effects of both forms of vitamin D cannot be drawn at this time.

VITAMIN D ASSAY METHODOLOGY

Serum 25(OH)D comprises of $25(OH)D_2$ and $25(OH)D_3$. In US and Canada, the assay used measures both $25(OH)D_2$ and $25(OH)D_3$ to give a total 25(OH)D level, whereas in Europe the commercial assays measure only $25(OH)D_3$ since only vitamin D_3 is used [14]. It is important to note that different 25(OH)D assay methods have been developed over the years, with each assay having inherent variability. Due to the shifts in assay performance over time, one needs to recognize the limitations in making direct comparisons among studies, such as comparing 25(OH)D levels reported in the NHANES III (1984 to 1994) with those from NHANES 2000 to 2006.

VITAMIN D SAFETY AND TOXICITY

The benefit of increasing vitamin D intake through dietary or oral supplementation needs to be balanced against the risk of hypervitaminosis D, as there is a U-shaped curve between vitamin D and all-cause mortality [14, 27, 72]. The 2011 IOM report sets the tolerable upper level of vitamin D intake to 4000 IU/day for ages 9 and older. This upper level of vitamin D intake is not intended as a target intake but a level above which the potential risk of adverse effects may increase. The IOM derived the conservative upper level of vitamin D intake with hypercalcemia as the indicator of acute vitamin D toxicity.

Although the body obtains vitamin D from cutaneous synthesis as well as oral vitamin D intake, vitamin D toxicity mainly results from excessive oral vitamin D ingestion. Excessive oral vitamin D intake from dietary or oral supplementation leads to increased intestinal absorption of calcium and bone resorption, resulting in acute and/or chronic hypercalcemia. Acute hypercalcemia can manifest as anorexia, cardiac arrhythmias and polyuria (that can lead to renal impairment). Chronic hypercalcemia over time leads to calcium-phosphate deposition in the vasculature, resulting in vascular calcification and stiffness [44].

Skin-produced vitamin D is generally considered safe as vitamin D toxicity is prevented by the breakdown of excess vitamin D_3 formed from prolonged sun exposure [5]. However, there is much concern over the risk of skin cancer associated with excessive sun exposure, as the spectra of UVB for vitamin D synthesis may cause skin cancer [27]. The level of sun exposure sufficient to maintain adequate vitamin D levels without increasing the risk of skin cancer is difficult to determine due to the variable UVB intensity with latitude, altitude, time of day and year. The amount of vitamin D_3 synthesized varies with the skin melanin content with fair-skinned persons being able to photosynthesize vitamin D_3 most effectively while also having the highest risk of skin cancer. In addition, the other variables that were mentioned earlier such as cultural difference in clothing and reduced synthesis of 7-dehydrocholesterol with aging make it difficult to put forth a standard recommendation on sun exposure for the general population.

It was initially thought that vitamin D toxicity involved an increase in the active metabolite $1,25(OH)_2D$, but some animal studies and human case reports of vitamin D intoxication found individuals with elevated $25(OH)D$ but normal $1,25(OH)_2D$ [15]. Hence, serum $25(OH)D$ but not $1,25(OH)_2D$ is used as a biomarker for vitamin D toxicity. However, the $25(OH)D$ threshold at which vitamin D toxicity occurs in humans is less well-defined [14]. Vitamin D toxicity has been reported within a wide range of serum $25(OH)D$ levels, from 24 to 600 ng/mL. The IOM committee set the upper limit of $25(OH)D$ at 50 ng/mL due to: (1) bone health benefit is achieved at 20 ng/mL for 97.5% of the population, and (2) data related to all-cause mortality, chronic disease risk and falls suggest that adverse events may occur with serum $25(OH)D$ levels greater than 30 ng/mL, ranging up to 50 ng/mL.

CONCLUSION

While there is undisputable scientific evidence to support the role of vitamin D and calcium in maintaining bone health, the emerging role of VDR in other health outcomes such as infection, cancer and cardiovascular disease has generated much interest in the potential use of vitamin D supplementation to manage these disorders. At present, available studies on vitamin D for these conditions have shown mixed results, requiring further research to demonstrate its efficacies.

Current DRI recommendations on vitamin D intake are derived from studies on bone health, with $25(OH)D$ as a surrogate marker of exposure. As the prevalence and risk factors for vitamin D deficiency are increasingly recognized, the impetus to administer vitamin D supplement to as many people as possible needs to be balanced against the risk of potential toxicity associated with the lack of monitoring. Therefore, the practice of giving standard doses of vitamin D supplement may need to be assessed in light of the optimal $25(OH)D$ levels, to derive maximal protective benefits from this readily available and affordable vitamin without its undue toxicities.

REFERENCES

[1]   DeLuca HF. Overview of general physiologic features and functions of vitamin D. Am J Clin Nutr 2004; 80: 1689S-1696S.

[2]   Holick MF, Chen TC. Vitamin D deficiency: a worldwide problem with health consequences. Am J Clin Nutr 2008; 87: 1080S-1086S.

[3]   Wolpowitz D, Gilchrest BA. The vitamin D questions: how much do you need and how should you get it? J Am Acad Dermatol 2006; 54:301-317.

[4]   Holick MF. Vitamin D: importance in the prevention of cancers, type 1 diabetes, heart disease, and osteoporosis. Am J Clin Nutr 2004; 79:362-371.

[5]   Holick MF. Sunlight and vitamin D for bone health and prevention of autoimmune diseases, cancers, and cardiovascular disease. Am J Clin Nutr 2004; 80:1678S-1688S.

[6]   Holick MF. Vitamin D deficiency. N Engl J Med 2007; 357:266-281.

[7]   Liu S, Gupta A, Quarles LD. Emerging role of fibroblast growth factor 23 in a bone-kidney axis regulating systemic phosphate homeostasis and extracellular matrix mineralization. Curr Opin Nephrol Hypertens 2007; 16:329-335.

[8]   Jones G. Expanding role for vitamin D in chronic kidney disease: importance of blood 25-OH-D levels and extra-renal 1alpha-hydroxylase in the classical and nonclassical actions of 1alpha,25-dihydroxyvitamin D(3). Semin Dial 2007; 20:316-324.

[9]   Bikle D. Nonclassic actions of vitamin D. J Clin Endocrinol Metab 2009; 94:26-34.

[10]   Heaney RP. Vitamin D in health and disease. Clin J Am Soc Nephrol 2008; 3:1535-1541.

[11]   Hewison M, Burke F, Evans KN, *et al.* Extra-renal 25-hydroxyvitamin D3-1alpha-hydroxylase in human health and disease. J Steroid Biochem Mol Biol 2007; 103:316-321.

[12]   Holick MF. The vitamin D deficiency pandemic and consequences for nonskeletal health: mechanisms of action. Mol Aspects Med 2008; 29:361-368.

[13]   Maalouf NM. The noncalciotropic actions of vitamin D: recent clinical developments. Curr Opin Nephrol Hypertens 2008; 17:408-415.

[14]   Institute of Medicine 2011. Dietary reference intakes for calcium and vitamin D. In: Ross AC, Taylor CL, Yaktine AL, Del Valle HB, editors. Washing, DC: The National Academies Press, 2011.

[15] Jones G. Pharmacokinetics of vitamin D toxicity. Am J Clin Nutr 2008; 88:582S-586S.

[16] Institute of Medicine 1997. Dietary reference intakes for calcium, phosphorus, magnesium, vitamin D, and fluoride. Washington, DC: The National Academies Press, 1997.

[17] Holick MF. The D-lemma: to screen or not to screen for 25-hydroxyvitamin D concentrations. Clin Chem 2010; 56:729-731.

[18] Sai AJ, Walters RW, Fang X, Gallagher JC. Relationship between vitamin D, parathyroid hormone, and bone health. J Clin Endocrinol Metab 2011; 96:E436-446.

[19] Looker AC, Johnson CL, Lacher DA, Pfeiffer CM, Schleicher RL, Sempos CT, Vitamin D status: United States, 2001-2006. In: Statistics NCfH, editor. Hyattsville, MD: DHHS, 2011: 1-7.

[20] Malabanan A, Veronikis IE, Holick MF. Redefining vitamin D insufficiency. Lancet 1998; 351:805-806.

[21] Bischoff-Ferrari HA, Dietrich T, Orav EJ, Dawson-Hughes B. Positive association between 25-hydroxy vitamin D levels and bone mineral density: a population-based study of younger and older adults. Am J Med 2004; 116:634-639.

[22] Bischoff-Ferrari HA, Willett WC, Wong JB, et al. Prevention of nonvertebral fractures with oral vitamin D and dose dependency: a meta-analysis of randomized controlled trials. Arch Intern Med 2009; 169:551-561.

[23] Bischoff-Ferrari HA, Willett WC, Wong JB, Giovannucci E, Dietrich T, Dawson-Hughes B. Fracture prevention with vitamin D supplementation: a meta-analysis of randomized controlled trials. JAMA 2005; 293:2257-2264.

[24] Jackson RD, LaCroix AZ, Gass M, et al. Calcium plus vitamin D supplementation and the risk of fractures. N Engl J Med 2006; 354:669-683.

[25] Avenell A, Gillespie WJ, Gillespie LD, O'Connell D. Vitamin D and vitamin D analogues for preventing fractures associated with involutional and post-menopausal osteoporosis. Cochrane Database Syst Rev 2009:CD000227.

[26] van den Bergh JP, Bours SP, van Geel TA, Geusens PP. Optimal use of vitamin D when treating osteoporosis. Curr Osteoporos Rep 2011; 9:36-42.

[27] Brannon PM, Yetley EA, Bailey RL, Picciano MF. Overview of the conference "Vitamin D and Health in the 21st Century: an Update". Am J Clin Nutr 2008; 88:483S-490S.

[28] Bischoff-Ferrari HA, Dawson-Hughes B, Willett WC, et al. Effect of Vitamin D on falls: a meta-analysis. Jama 2004; 291:1999-2006.

[29] Melamed ML, Michos ED, Post W, Astor B. 25-hydroxyvitamin D levels and the risk of mortality in the general population. Arch Intern Med 2008; 168:1629-1637.

[30] Autier P, Gandini S. Vitamin D supplementation and total mortality: a meta-analysis of randomized controlled trials. Arch Intern Med 2007; 167:1730-1737.

[31] Giovannucci E. Can vitamin D reduce total mortality? Arch Intern Med 2007; 167:1709-1710.

[32] Dobnig H, Pilz S, Scharnagl H, et al. Independent association of low serum 25-hydroxyvitamin d and 1,25-dihydroxyvitamin d levels with all-cause and cardiovascular mortality. Arch Intern Med 2008; 168:1340-1349.

[33] Ginde AA, Scragg R, Schwartz RS, Camargo CA, Jr. Prospective study of serum 25-hydroxyvitamin D level, cardiovascular disease mortality, and all-cause mortality in older U.S. adults. J Am Geriatr Soc 2009; 57:1595-1603.

[34] Zittermann A, Koerfer R. Vitamin D in the prevention and treatment of coronary heart disease. Curr Opin Clin Nutr Metab Care 2008; 11:752-757.

[35] Levin A, Li YC. Vitamin D and its analogues: do they protect against cardiovascular disease in patients with kidney disease? Kidney Int 2005; 68:1973-1981.

[36] Nemerovski CW, Dorsch MP, Simpson RU, Bone HG, Aaronson KD, Bleske BE. Vitamin D and cardiovascular disease. Pharmacotherapy 2009; 29:691-708.

[37] Li YC, Qiao G, Uskokovic M, Xiang W, Zheng W, Kong J. Vitamin D: a negative endocrine regulator of the renin-angiotensin system and blood pressure. J Steroid Biochem Mol Biol 2004; 89-90:387-392.

[38] Pittas AG, Chung M, Trikalinos T, et al. Systematic review: Vitamin D and cardiometabolic outcomes. Ann Intern Med 2010; 152:307-314.

[39] Achinger SG, Ayus JC. The role of vitamin D in left ventricular hypertrophy and cardiac function. Kidney Int Suppl 2005:S37-42.

[40] Shoji T, Shinohara K, Kimoto E, et al. Lower risk for cardiovascular mortality in oral 1alpha-hydroxy vitamin D3 users in a haemodialysis population. Nephrol Dial Transplant 2004; 19:179-184.

[41] Cunningham J, Zehnder D. New vitamin D analogs and changing therapeutic paradigms. Kidney Int 2011; 79:702-707.

[42] Teng M, Wolf M, Lowrie E, Ofsthun N, Lazarus JM, Thadhani R. Survival of patients undergoing hemodialysis with paricalcitol or calcitriol therapy. N Engl J Med 2003; 349:446-456.

[43]   Wu-Wong JR. Potential for vitamin D receptor agonists in the treatment of cardiovascular disease. Br J Pharmacol 2009; 158:395-412.

[44]   Razzaque MS. The dualistic role of vitamin D in vascular calcifications. Kidney Int 2011; 79:708-714.

[45]   IARC. Vitamin D and Cancer. In: Reports IWG, editor. Lyon, France: International Agency for Research on Cancer 2008.

[46]   Holick MF. Vitamin D and sunlight: strategies for cancer prevention and other health benefits. Clin J Am Soc Nephrol 2008; 3:1548-1554.

[47]   Trump DL, Deeb KK, Johnson CS. Vitamin D: considerations in the continued development as an agent for cancer prevention and therapy. Cancer J 2010; 16:1-9.

[48]   Giovannucci E. The epidemiology of vitamin D and cancer incidence and mortality: a review (United States). Cancer Causes Control 2005; 16:83-95.

[49]   Matthews D, LaPorta E, Zinser GM, Narvaez CJ, Welsh J. Genomic vitamin D signaling in breast cancer: Insights from animal models and human cells. J Steroid Biochem Mol Biol 2010; 121:362-367.

[50]   Yin L, Grandi N, Raum E, Haug U, Arndt V, Brenner H. Meta-analysis: serum vitamin D and breast cancer risk. Eur J Cancer 2010; 46:2196-2205.

[51]   Rheem DS, Baylink DJ, Olafsson S, Jackson CS, Walter MH. Prevention of colorectal cancer with vitamin D. Scand J Gastroenterol 2010; 45:775-784.

[52]   Wactawski-Wende J, Kotchen JM, Anderson GL, *et al.* Calcium plus vitamin D supplementation and the risk of colorectal cancer. N Engl J Med 2006; 354:684-696.

[53]   Lappe JM, Travers-Gustafson D, Davies KM, Recker RR, Heaney RP. Vitamin D and calcium supplementation reduces cancer risk: results of a randomized trial. Am J Clin Nutr 2007; 85:1586-1591.

[54]   Bikle DD. Vitamin D and the immune system: role in protection against bacterial infection. Curr Opin Nephrol Hypertens 2008; 17:348-352.

[55]   Adams JS, Hewison M. Update in vitamin D. J Clin Endocrinol Metab 2010; 95:471-478.

[56]   Hewison M. Vitamin D and the immune system: new perspectives on an old theme. Endocrinol Metab Clin North Am 2010; 39:365-379, table of contents.

[57]   Verstuyf A, Carmeliet G, Bouillon R, Mathieu C. Vitamin D: a pleiotropic hormone. Kidney Int 2010; 78:140-145.

[58]   White JH. Vitamin D signaling, infectious diseases, and regulation of innate immunity. Infect Immun 2008; 76:3837-3843.

[59]   Liu PT, Stenger S, Li H, *et al.* Toll-like receptor triggering of a vitamin D-mediated human antimicrobial response. Science 2006; 311:1770-1773.

[60]   Yamshchikov AV, Desai NS, Blumberg HM, Ziegler TR, Tangpricha V. Vitamin D for treatment and prevention of infectious diseases: a systematic review of randomized controlled trials. Endocr Pract 2009; 15:438-449.

[61]   Stechschulte SA, Kirsner RS, Federman DG. Vitamin D: bone and beyond, rationale and recommendations for supplementation. Am J Med 2009; 122:793-802.

[62]   Baz-Hecht M, Goldfine AB. The impact of vitamin D deficiency on diabetes and cardiovascular risk. Curr Opin Endocrinol Diabetes Obes 2010; 17:113-119.

[63]   Zipitis CS, Akobeng AK. Vitamin D supplementation in early childhood and risk of type 1 diabetes: a systematic review and meta-analysis. Arch Dis Child 2008; 93:512-517.

[64]   Hypponen E, Laara E, Reunanen A, Jarvelin MR, Virtanen SM. Intake of vitamin D and risk of type 1 diabetes: a birth-cohort study. Lancet 2001; 358:1500-1503.

[65]   Hughes DA, Norton R. Vitamin D and respiratory health. Clin Exp Immunol 2009; 158:20-25.

[66]   Lee P, Nair P, Eisman JA, Center JR. Vitamin D deficiency in the intensive care unit: an invisible accomplice to morbidity and mortality? Intensive Care Med 2009; 35:2028-2032.

[67]   Pittas AG, Lau J, Hu FB, Dawson-Hughes B. The role of vitamin D and calcium in type 2 diabetes. A systematic review and meta-analysis. J Clin Endocrinol Metab 2007; 92:2017-2029.

[68]   Wagner CL, Greer FR. Prevention of rickets and vitamin D deficiency in infants, children, and adolescents. Pediatrics 2008; 122:1142-1152.

[69]   Armas LA, Hollis BW, Heaney RP. Vitamin D2 is much less effective than vitamin D3 in humans. J Clin Endocrinol Metab 2004; 89:5387-5391.

[70]   Houghton LA, Vieth R. The case against ergocalciferol (vitamin D2) as a vitamin supplement. Am J Clin Nutr 2006; 84:694-697.

[71]   Holick MF, Biancuzzo RM, Chen TC, *et al.* Vitamin D2 is as effective as vitamin D3 in maintaining circulating concentrations of 25-hydroxyvitamin D. J Clin Endocrinol Metab 2008; 93:677-681.

[72]   Ross AC, Manson JE, Abrams SA, *et al.* The 2011 report on dietary reference intakes for calcium and vitamin D from the Institute of Medicine: what clinicians need to know. J Clin Endocrinol Metab; 96:53-58.

CHAPTER 5

Vitamin D Analogs Currently on the Market and in Development

Gui-Dong Zhu[*]

Cancer Research, GPRD, Abbott Laboratories, 100 Abbott Park Rd, Abbott Park, IL 60064, USA

Abstract: Since the discovery of $1\alpha,25$-dihydroxyvitamin D_3 (calcitriol), the active form of vitamin D, in early 1970s, research in the vitamin D endocrine system has received increasing attention. The biological actions of calcitriol have subsequently been shown to extend well beyond its classical functions in calcium homeostasis to include immune and angiogenesis, cell cycle, apoptosis, as well as endocrine regulations. While calcitriol demonstrates significant efficacy in treating hyperproliferative disorders (*e.g.* cancer and psoriasis), immune dysfunction (autoimmune diseases), and endocrine disorders (*e.g.* hyperparathyroidism), its calcemic activity limits a broader therapeutic application of this vitamin D hormone. The medicinal chemistry efforts have primarily been directed to the differentiation of the desired therapeutic activity from the toxic episodic effects. More than three thousands vitamin D derivatives have been synthesized and some of them showed separation of the beneficial activities from calcemic effects. Nine vitamin D compounds have been approved in the United States, Japan or Europe for a number of indications. This review attempts to serve as a progress report for the vitamin D analogs currently on the market and in clinical development.

Keywords: Alfacalcidol, calcidiol, calcipotriol (dovonex, daivonex, psorcutan), calcitriol, doxercalciterol (hectorol), eldecalcitol, elocalcitol, falecalcitriol (hornel/fulstan), maxacalcitol (oxarol), paricalcitol (zemplar), seocalcitol, tacalcitol (bonalfa, curatoderm).

INTRODUCTION

Vitamin D is a generic term for a family of secosteroids that were discovered and associated with bone health as early as in 1922. Since the characterization of its active form, $1\alpha,25$-dihydroxyvitamin D_3 $(1,25(OH)_2D_3)$ in 1970, interest in vitamin D research has been kept at an enormously high level and the pace of research seemed to be accelerated in the past decade. Vitamin D has emerged as a universal regulator in a variety of cells of higher animals and involved in a host of biological functions [1]. The vitamin D receptor is now known to be present in over 35 tissues. Vitamin D is believed to be critical for a number of non-classical physiological functions, including DNA repair, reduction on inflammation, and promotion on the death of potentially malignant cells. The ever broadening spectrum of vitamin D activities warrants therapeutic applications of the vitamin D hormone for the treatment of hyperproliferative disorders (*e.g.* psoriasis, cancer), immune disfunction, endocrine disorders, and heart disease, all systems that have vitamin D receptor (VDR).

As mentioned in previous chapters and now illustrated with chemical structures in Fig. **1**, the natural vitamin D is primarily produced in skin upon ultraviolet irradiation of 7-dehydrocholesterol or directly absorbed from the diet. The reaction in skin is believed to be a photochemical process, first generating previtamin D_3 which spontaneously isomerizes to vitamin D_3. The initially formed 6-cis form of vitamin D_3 is in quick equilibrium with its trans form with the latter predominating.

A plasma protein, namely vitamin D-binding protein (DBP), subsequently binds and transports vitamin D_3 to liver where it interacts with a cytochrome P450 enzyme 25-hydroxlase, generating 25-hydroxyvitamin D_3 $(25(OH)D_3)$. $25(OH)D_3$, as the major circulating form of vitamin D in serum, does not seem to have physiological functions on its own and is further transported to kidney where it is metabolized by 25-hydroxy-D-1α-hydroxylase (CYP27B1) to form $1,25(OH)_2D_3$, the physiologically active hormonal form. The hormone $1,25(OH)_2D_3$ can bind to DBP and is then transported to targeted organs including bone, intestine, and kidney.

*Address correspondence Gui-Dong Zhu: Cancer Research, GPRD, Abbott Laboratories, 100 Abbott Park Rd., Abbott Park , IL , 60064, USA; E-mail: gui-dong.zhu@abbott.com

$1,25(OH)_2D_3$, also called calcitriol, regulates the concentration of calcium and phosphate in the bloodstream, promoting the healthy mineralization, growth and remodeling of bone, and the prevention of hypocalcemic tetany. Vitamin D insufficiency can result in thin, brittle, or misshapen bones, while sufficiency prevents rickets in children and osteomalacia in adults. Calcitriol mediates its biological effects by binding to the VDR, which is primarily located in the nuclei of target cells. The binding of calcitriol to the VDR leads to modulation of gene expression of VDR target genes including transport proteins involved in calcium absorption in the intestine.

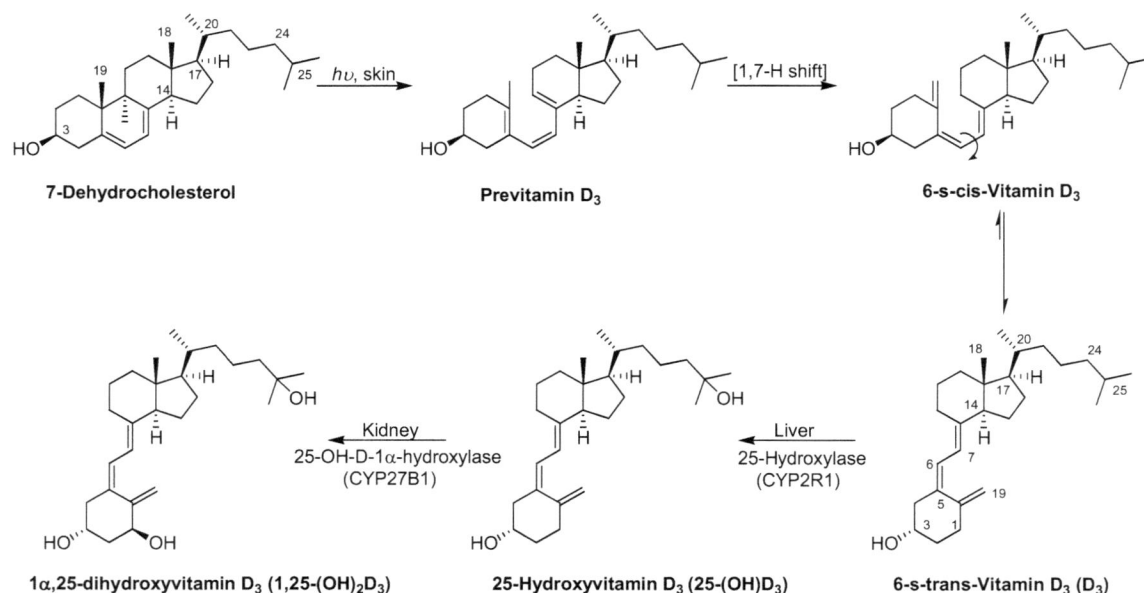

Figure 1: Biosynthesis of vitamin D.

The blood calcitriol level is tightly regulated by feedback control of both synthetic and catabolic pathways as described in previous chapters. In response to either low serum calcium or phosphate, the parathyroid gland secrets more parathyroid hormone (PTH), which stimulates the transcription of CYP27B1, increasing the level of $1,25(OH)D_3$. Encoded by the CYP24A1 gene, the mitochondrial 1,25-dihydroxyvitamin D_3 24-hydroxylase is a member of the cytochrome P450 superfamily of enzymes. CYP24A1 is a monooxygenase which catalyzes the 24-hydroxlation of $1,25(OH)_2D_3$ and break down the active vitamin D hormone. Documented evidence has linked low levels of vitamin D to a higher incidence of cancer and worse survival. Overexpression of CYP24A1 results in increased metabolism of vitamin D, leading to increased incidence and recurrence of lung cancer [2]. The studies from University of Michigan Comprehensive Cancer suggest that levels of CYP24A1 were elevated as much as 50 times in lung adenocarcinoma relative to normal lung tissues. The high level of CYP24A1 is also linked to an increased probability of more aggressive tumor and decreased survival rate. So, CYP24A1, as well as its encoded enzyme, may be useful to serve as a personalized approach to prevent lung cancer from recurrence and spreading after surgery [2]. Blocking the activity of CYP24A1 in combination with high dose of vitamin D could potentially be an attractive approach for prevention or treatment of lung cancer.

The increasing body of medicinal chemistry efforts has been directed toward the development of clinically useful vitamin D drugs for a diverse set of disease indications. More than three thousand of vitamin D analogs have been synthesized and evaluated [3]. Major attention has focused on dissociation of a beneficial biological activity (*e.g.* cell differentiation) from the major toxic episodic effects such as hypercalcemia and hyperphosphatemia. The crystal structure of a ligand-binding domain of VDR in complex with vitamin D analog [4, 5] has revealed that the binding pocket for the vitamin D hormone is rather large. It would be relatively challenging to structurally design targeted analogs with specific physiological functions. It also seems to be true that the vitamin D analogs with significant difference in biological activity do not display marked change in the binding mode in the X-ray structure of VDR. These distinctive characteristics make the medicinal chemistry effort in the vitamin D research unique. In most of cases, the selected clinical compounds emerged as a result of evaluating from cell culture to direct animal and clinical studies.

While an extensive review on the structure-activity relationship (SAR) of the secosteroid is beyond the scope of this chapter, Fig. **2** highlights some of the more common structural modifications that tempt to bring in improved activity for cell differentiation with reduced calcemic functions. The analogs with C-20 epi side chain, the C-22 incorporated oxygen and the one carbon homologated C-26,27 methyl group, all discovered at Leo Pharmaceutical, frequently display up to two logs of higher activity than $1,25(OH)_2D_3$ in inhibition of cellular growth. More importantly, these vitamin D derivatives demonstrate less calcemic activity *in vivo* as compared to the parent compound.

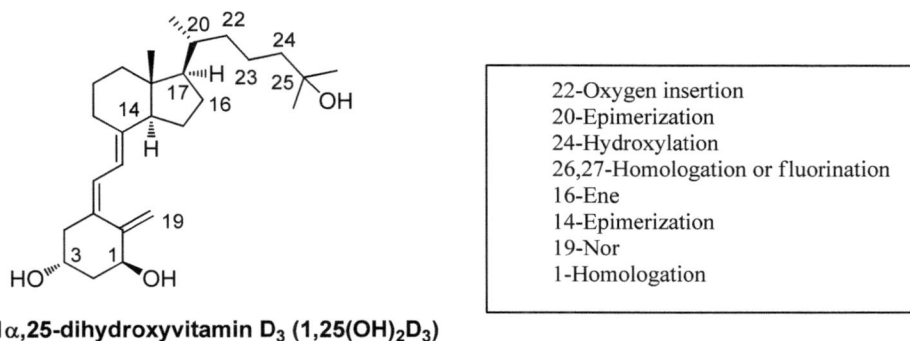

22-Oxygen insertion
20-Epimerization
24-Hydroxylation
26,27-Homologation or fluorination
16-Ene
14-Epimerization
19-Nor
1-Homologation

1α,25-dihydroxyvitamin D₃ (1,25(OH)₂D₃)

Figure 2: Common structural modifications that showed improved cell differentiating with reduced calcemic activities.

Insertion of a double bond unsaturation between the C16 and C17 carbons (16-ene), in conjunction with or without other structural changes, is another common modification that leads to differentiation of the beneficial cell differentiation activity from the episodic hypercalcemic response. For example, a simple 16-ene analog of $1,25-(OH)_2D_3$ is between 10-100 times more potent in inhibiting clonal growth of a number of myeloid leukemia cell lines and 7 times more potent in inducing cellular differentiation while maintaining similar hypercalcemic activity to that of its parent compound [6]. A fortuitous result also showed that incorporating either C23-ene or –yne functionality into the side chain of $1,25(OH)_2D_3$ significantly reduced the hypercalcemic activity of these analogs with the latter being 55-fold less hypercalcemic compared to that of calcitriol. Despite of synthetic challenges, it is generally accepted that certain modifications to the A-ring lead to a pronounced separation of anti-proliferative activity from its classical function for calcium homeostasis. One of the examples for these modifications includes the removal of the C-19 exomethylene (19-nor), resulting in great activity in inducing cell differentiation of malignant cells with little or no hyprcalcemic activity. Posner's group has demonstrated that one carbon homologation at the C-1 position (1-hydroxymethyl) of the A-ring is detrimental to its hypercalcemic but cell differentiating activity. A combination of this modification with a 16-ene anti-proliferative moiety, along with C-24 fluorination and 26,27-homologation to block catabolism, led to an extremely potent inhibitor of multistage skin tumorigenesis with nearly 80-100 fold less hypercalciuric activity than $1,25(OH)_2D_3$ [7]. The SAR on the 14-epimerization, however, is somehow controversial, though more than 10-fold enhancement in antiproliferative action and up to 400-fold reduction in calcemic effects have been reported for this modification incorporated with a 23-yne [7].

The vitamin D endocrine system has provided novel approaches for the treatment and prevention of a wide range of diseases. More than nine vitamin D based compounds have been approved for clinical uses, with many more in development. Table **1** lists the major therapeutic applications of the natural vitamin D hormone and its analogs. Most of the indications including cardiovascular disease [8], kidney disease [9, 10], hyperproliferative disorders [11, 12], and thrombosis [13], along with clinically approved vitamin derivatives, have been thoroughly covered by various review articles. An updated list of these compounds has been displayed in Table **2**, including the natural vitamin D_3 as a nutritional supplement.

Table 1: Common indications of vitamin D therapy

Indications	Representative Vitamin D Therapies	Causes	Potential Mechanism
Rickets Osteomalacia	Vitamin D, calcitriol Alfacalcidol, eldecalcitol (ED-71)	Nutrition, kidney failure, genetic disorders (*e.g.* CYP27B1 defects, VDR gene mutation)	Vitamin D is a regulator of calcium homeostasis, affecting bone remodeling
Kidney disease (Secondary hyperparathyroidism)	Calcitriol, paricalcitol, doxercalciferol, alfacalcidol, maxacalcitol, falecalcitriol	Renal osteodystrophy, decreased vitamin D hormone synthesis	Hypocalcemia stimulates the PTH synthesis and secretion
Psoriasis	Calcitriol, calcipotriol, maxacalcitol, tacalcitol	An autoimmune disease, increased keratinocyte hyperproliferation	VDR has been found in keratinocytes, sebocytes and dermal papilla cells. Keratinocyctes proliferation is suppressed by $1,25(OH)_2D_3$ *in vitro*
Cardiovascular disease	Vitamin D, calcitriol, paricalcitol	Vitamin D deficiency, renal failure	VDR found in vascular smooth muscle and cardiomyocytes, and involved in renin-angiotensin regulation and coagulation response modulation
Prostate cancer, breast cancer, colon cancer, leukemia	Many analogs including calcitriol, paricalcitol, doxercalciferol, elocalcitol, EB1089 in clinical trials, no marketed drug yet	Increased cell proliferation and decreased cell differentiation	VDR may be involved in cell cycle regulation and cell proliferation inhibition

Table 2: Selected vitamin D analogs currently on the market and in development

Generic name (Trade Name)	Compound Name	Structure	Company	Indications and Development Status
Calcidiol Didrogyl Hidroferol	25-Hydroxyvitamin D_3		Upjohn Organon Faes Farma	Renal osteodystrophy, osteoporosis, rickets and others
Alfacalcidol (Alfarol, One-Alpha, On-Alfa)	1α-Hydroxyvitamin D_3		Chugai Leo/Teijin Leo	Rickets, osteomalacia, osteoporosis, launched in Japan in 1981
Calcitriol (Rocaltrol, Calcijex, Decostriol)	1α,25-Dihydroxyvitamin D_3 (calcitriol)		Roche Abbott Mibe, Jesalis	Rickets, osteomalacia, secondary hyperparathyroidism, launched

Table 2: cont....

Doxercalciterol (Hectorol)	1α-Hydroxyvitamin D₂		Bone Care International (Genzyme, Sanofi)	Secondary hyperparathyroidism (launched in the US in 1999)
Paricalcitol (Zemplar)	1α,25-Dihydroxyvitamin D₂		Abbott	Secondary hyperparathyroidism (launched in the US in 1998)
Calcipotriol (Dovonex, Daivonex, Psorcutan)	24(R)-1α,24-Dihydroxy-22-ene-25-ethylene-26,27-nor-vitamin D₃ (calcipotriene, MC-903)		Leo	Psoriasis vulgaris (Pso, launched in Europe in 1991)
Seocalcitol	1α,26-Dihydroxy-22,24-diene-25-homo-26-diethylvitamin D₃ (EB1089)		Leo	Psoriasis and hepatocellular carcinoma (discontinued as single agent)
Tacalcitol (Bonalfa, Curatoderm)	24(R)-1α,24-Dihydroxyvitamin D₃		Teijin Institute for Bio-Medical Research	Psoriasis vulgaris (Pso, launched in Japan in 1993)
Maxacalcitol (Oxarol)	1α,25-Dihydroxy-22-oxavitamin D₃ (OCT)		Chugai	Secondary hyperparathyroidism (launched in 2000 in Japan) Psoriasis vulgaris (Pso, launched in 2001 in Japan)
Falecalcitriol (Hornel/Fulstan)	26,26,26,27,27,27-Hexafluoro-1α,25-dihydroxyvitamin D₃		Taisho /Sumitomo, Kissei	Secondary hyperparathyroidism (launched in Japan in 2001)

Table 2: cont....

Eldecalcitol	1α,25-Dihydroxy-2β-(3-hydroxypropoxy)-vitamin D$_3$ (ED-71)		Chugai	Osteoporosis (NDA filed in 2009)
Elocalcitol	(23E)-1α-Fluoro-25-hydroxy-16,17,23,24-tetrahydro-26,27-bishomo-20-epivitamin D$_3$ (BXL-628)		BioXell SpA	Benign PH Overactive Bladder (OAB), Terminated in April 2009
CTA018	24-tert-Butylsulfonyl-16,23-diene-1α,25-dihydroxy-25,26,27-Norvitamin D$_3$		Cytochroma	Secondary hyperparathyroidism (Phase II)
2MD	2-Methylene-19-nor-(20S)-1α,25-dihydroxyvitamin D$_3$, 2MD		Deltanoid	Osteoporosis (Phase II)

The remainder of the chapter will focus on vitamin D supplement and the vitamin D analogs currently on the market and in development. It will be apparent to the readers that a large number of "designer" vitamin D analogues synthesized in the past couple of decades display dramatically reduced calcemic activity *in vitro* while retaining other desired activities. Unfortunately, discrepancies exist between experimental data and clinical studies. None of these compounds are truly non-calcaemic in clinical setting. For any new vitamin D analog, head-to-head studies against established treatments may be needed to demonstrate a clear clinical edge.

VITAMIN D SUPPLEMENT

Although other chapters have provided many details on the subject of vitamin D supplement, for the completion of the discussion on the applications of vitamin D and its analogs, some key points are reinterated in this chapter.

Vitamin D$_3$ is known to be essential to maintain bone health and is the most widely used supplement in the vitamin D endocrine system. Appropriate dietary vitamin supplementation is critical in preventing vitamin D deficiency children rickets and adult osteomalacia. Based on a review of almost 1,000 studies and testimony from scientists and others, Institute of Medicine of the National Academies released an updated Dietary Reference Intake (DRI) allowance for vitamin D on November 2010. Under the new guidelines, the recommended vitamin D intake is 600 IU/d (15 μg/d) for infants, children and adult male and female subjects up to age 70. For men and women aged over 70, the recommended dose was set at 800 IU/d (20 µg/d). The DRI allowance for calcium is 700 milligrams per day for children aged 1 through 3, 1,000 milligrams for children aged 4 through 8, and 1300 mg for children and adolescents aged 9 through 18 [14]. In conjunction with the updated DRI for vitamin D, 1000 milligrams daily intake of calcium is recommended for most adults aged 19 through 50 and for men up to 70 years. For women aged 51 and older, and for both men and women aged 71 and older, 1200 milligrams a day of calcium is enough. Taking in too much calcium from supplements has been linked with kidney stones, while excessive vitamin D consumption can damage the kidneys and heart [15].

The major form of vitamin D supplement includes a mixture of vitamin D_2 (ergocalciferol) and vitamin D_3 (cholecalciferol). Though pharmacopoeias have officially regarded these two forms as equivalent and interchangeable, an emerging body of evidence suggests that vitamin D_3 is the more potent form of vitamin D and should be recommended as a nutrient suitable for supplementation or fortification [16]. Vitamin D status is commonly determined for 25(OH)D through a blood test. A level at less than 20 ng/mL is usually defined as deficiency and less than 5 ng/mL as severe deficiency, though this guideline is being re-examined. Vitamin D insufficiency is generally considered to be widespread, and up to 50 percent of patients seen in routine clinical practice have vitamin D levels below the optimal range. Level of vitamin D is crucial to bone development and bone health, in particular to children. An exposure of above 200 ng/mL in blood level is commonly considered to be toxic, but taking several thousand IU daily will not bring blood levels of 25(OH)D even close to that threshold. Hackman *et al.* compared the efficacy and safety of a 10-day, high-dose (50,000 IU daily for 10 days) *vs.* a 3-month, continuous low-dose (3000 IU daily for 30 days, followed by 1000 IU daily for 60 days) oral cholecalciferol regimen in a randomized and open-label clinical trial enrolling 59 vitamin D deficient patients (serum 25(OH)D ≤50 nmol/L) [17]. Both groups also received calcium citrate 500 mg daily. A similar increase in mean serum 25(OH)D and incidents in hypercalciuria (urine calcium >7.5 mmol/day) and vitamin D toxicity (25(OH)D >200 nmol/L) during the study was observed. Thus, the high-dose regimen may be an effective approach to treat patients with vitamin D deficiency.

The functions of vitamin D appear to extend well beyond bone health to include, for example, immune system regulation and anti-proliferative effects on cells. Through retroanalysis of a large volume of clinical trials with vitamin D supplements, it has been observed that higher serum exposure of vitamin D offers significant benefits for a range of human diseases and for cancer chemoprevention in particular. Vitamin D inadequacy in early life is linked to an increasing risk of bone disease, autoimmune disease, and implicated in certain cancers later in life. Although other chapters have covered these subjects in details, it is worth emphasizing here some of the particularly promising applications of vitamin D.

One of these is the link between lower levels of vitamin D and risk of cancer *via* epidemiological studies [18]. An association between vitamin D status (as evaluated by serum 25(OH)D levels) with breast and colon cancer but less likely with prostate cancer was reported in many studies [19- 21]. According to a report presented by Alisa Huston at the American Society of Bone and Mineral Research (October 16, 2010), an intriguing correlation between vitamin D deficiency and breast cancer was observed in a retrospective study of 224 women being treated for breast cancer at the URMC James P. Wilmot Cancer Center. In a separate study, it was found that the increased risk of colorectal cancer in the African American group is linked to their lower levels of vitamin D [22]. In a study enrolling 390 chronic lymphocytic leukemia (CLL) patients, researchers at Mayo Clinic also found that insufficient vitamin D levels in CLL patients were linked to cancer progression and death [23]. These findings have been confirmed by a separate study with 153 CLL patients who were followed for an average of 10 years. The World Health Organization conducted an extensive analysis of the epidemiological data on vitamin D and cancer and confirmed the observational studies that low 25(OH)D levels may be associated with increased risks for colorectal adenoma and cancer. However, a restrictive attitude should be taken regarding aggressive vitamin D supplementation or UVB exposure [24].

Retrospective studies have also linked poor vitamin D status with myocardial infarction (MI) and stroke. For example, a study published a few years ago reported that men with ≤15 ng/mL 25(OH)D had a relative risk of MI of 2.42 (95% CI; 1.53 - 3.84) compared with those with ≥30 ng/mL [25]. Several respective studies confirmed the correlations between increased mortality and severe vitamin D deficiency in normal subjects [26] and in patients with chronic kidney disease [27, 28]. More recently a systematic review of 52 clinical trials including 72 intervention groups and 6,290 patients on vitamin D supplementation revealed that negative logarithmic and linear correlations were found between 25(OH)D and PTH levels [29].

The impact of vitamin D status to immune regulation and multiple sclerosis was initially recognized from the observed geographical distribution of multiple sclerosis (MS). Areas with high sunlight exposure have a relatively low prevalence of multiple sclerosis and *vice versa*. Low plasma exposures of the principal vitamin D metabolite 25(OH)D were correlated with a high incidence of multiple sclerosis. Evidence suggests that vitamin D mediates a shift to a more anti-inflammatory immune response and also enhances regulatory T cell functionality [30]. Several retrospective studies have shown that vitamin D supplementation early in life reduces the subsequent risk of autoimmune Type I diabetes later in life [31, 32]. In an open-label randomized prospective 52 weeks trial that enrolled 49 patients with MS treated with escalating vitamin D doses up to 40,000 IU/day over 28 weeks followed by 10,000 IU/day for 12 weeks (plus 1,200 mg of calcium per day throughout the trial), treatment cohort as compared to placebo appeared to have fewer relapse events and a persistent reduction in T-cell proliferation, warranting a clinical trial design that adequately assess changes in clinical disease measures [33]. Lower serum 25(OH)D exposure is also associated with a substantially increased relapse rate in pediatric-onset multiple sclerosis or clinically isolated syndrome [34].

A survey of clinical trials of vitamin D supplementation published from 2000 to 2009 suggests that high normocalcemia (serum calcium levels that are high but fall within the normal reference range) may represent a more sensitive index of the long-term toxicity associated with vitamin D supplementation than hypercalcemia [35]. Therefore, efforts to chemoprevent diseases with vitamin D must consider the potential health risks associated with high normocalcemia.

ALFACALCIDOL

Alfacalcidol, a 1α-hydroxy analogue of vitamin D_3, is converted to the final active form calcitriol by 25-hydroxylation in the liver. Alfacalcidol was firstly approved for various indications at late 1970s and early 1980s and launched under main brand names of Alfarol, One-Alpha, and On-Alfa. Alfacalcidol was the first vitamin D analog to be indicated for the treatment of osteoporosis [36]. Alfacalcidol has been demonstrated in a number of clinical trials to maintain bone mineral density (BMD) in both postmenopausal osteoporosis and senile osteoporosis. It has a greater influence on BMD than plain vitamin D_3 does. In a multicenter trial, alfacalcidol reduced the incidence of vertebral fractures in postmenopausal women independent of the fracture history [37]. Tanizawa *et al.* showed in a retrospective study that alfacalcidol was helpful in reduction of hip fractures [38]. Alfacalcidol is considered to be an excellent partner for combination therapy to improve the antifracture efficacy, especially in elderly patients. A post-marketing survey of 13,550 patients given alfacalcidol ranging from 0.5 µg/day to 1 µg/day revealed minimal side effects including hypercalcemia (Ca^{2+} >11 mg/dL, 0.22% incidence) and increased urea nitrogen (0.15%) [39]. Only one case of kidney stone formation was found after 6 years on the alfacalcidol observational study of 8,093 patients.

Through a head-to-head comparison [40], alfacalcidol demonstrated superior therapeutic efficacy as compared to plain vitamin D_3 in glucocorticoid/inflammation-induced osteoporosis. Patients taking long term glucocorticoid (GC) therapy were included as matched pairs to receive randomly either 1 µg alfacalcidol plus 500 mg calcium per day (group A, n = 103) or 1000 IU vitamin D plus 500 mg calcium (group B, n = 101). A median increase of 2.4% in BMD at the lumbar spine was observed in the alfacalcidol group after a 3-year study *vs.* a loss of 0.8% in natural vitamin D_3 cohort (p <0.0001). The rate of patients with at least one new vertebral fracture was also significantly lower for the alfacalcidol group (9.7% *vs.* 24.8%). Consistent with the observed fracture rate, the alfacalcidol group showed a substantially larger decrease in back pain than the plain vitamin D group (p <0.0001). Generally, side effects in both groups were mild, and only 3 patients in the alfacalcidol group and 2 patients in the vitamin D group had moderate hypercalcemia.

Superior therapeutic efficacy was also observed for a combination regimen of alfacalcidol with alendronate as compared to plain vitamin D_3 in the same study [41]. The AAC-Trial (Alfacalcidol-Alendronate-Combined) enrolled 90 patients with established osteoporosis (57 women, 33 men) and included three treatment arms (alfacalcidol plus calcium, alendronate plus plain vitamin D and Ca^{2+}, and alendronate plus alfacalcidol and Ca^{2+}) over two years. The significantly higher lumbar spine and hip BMD increases were observed in the combined treatment group (p <0.001). The rate of patients with new vertebral and non-vertebral fractures after 2 years was 9 with alfacalcidol alone, 10 with alfacalcidol and plain vitamin D, and 2 in the group receiving alendronate plus alfacalidol (p <0.02). The alfacalcidol combination group also displayed a lower rate of falls and an earlier reduction of fracture.

In clinical situations characterized by a high rate of bone loss, including corticosteroid (CS)-induced osteoporosis, early postmenopausal bone loss, and organ transplant, alfacalcidol is particularly active compared to natural vitamin D_3 in improving bone turnover, increasing BMD, and reducing fracture rates [42]. Treatment with alfacalcidol 1 μg/day over 3 years fully prevented vertebral bone loss in women after the first year of menopause and spinal bone loss following treatment with high dose corticosteroid. In patients with established CS-induced osteoporosis with or without prevalent vertebral fractures, 1 μg/day of alfacalcidol given for 3 years increased lumbar spine density, reduced back pain, and showed a significant reduction in the rate of new vertebral fractures as compared to native vitamin D. In addition, when alfacalcidol and vitamin D_3 were compared in elderly women with radiologic evidence of vertebral fracture, fractional calcium absorption was increased after 3 months with alfacalcidol but was unchanged with vitamin D_3.

These data suggested that alfacalcidol is superior to the plain vitamin D for a number of indications and relatively safe with minimal adverse events. Alfacalcidol is also easier to be chemically synthesized and has demonstrated a relatively wider therapeutically window than calcitriol.

CALCITRIOL

Calcitriol is the endogenous active form of vitamin D_3. Calcitriol is marketed under various trade names including Rocaltrol-Nippon (Roche), Calcijex (Abbott) and Decostriol (Mibe, Jesalis). In additional to its traditional function for treatment and prevention of bone disease, calcitriol has demonstrated multiple potential clinical benefits for a variety of human diseases including cancer, immune-mediated diseases, cardiovascular diseases, and prostatic hypertrophy. However, these fascinating therapeutic possibilities suffer from drawbacks including relatively modest effects as stand-alone intervention at physiological concentration and hypercalcemia side effect at high dosage. Calcitriol is prescribed for treatment of hypocalcaemia and osteoporosis and prevention of corticosteroid-induced osteoporosis. The main adverse drug reaction associated with calcitriol therapy is hypercalcaemia with early symptoms such as nausea, vomiting, constipation, anorexia, apathy, headache, thirst, sweating, and/or polyuria.

Calcitriol was one of the earlier therapies for secondary hyperparathyroidism (SHPT, 2°HPT) that is common among patients with CKD. SHPT is associated with too much parathyroid hormone in the blood, resulting in huge amounts of calcium and phosphorus moving from bone into the blood, which weakens bones and makes bone disease highly prevalent in the CKD population. Also, the movement of calcium and phosphorus into the blood causes calcification of arteries, which may be linked to increased cardiovascular events and mortality even before CKD patients reach dialysis. Reduced renal mass in CKD patients leads to a decline in renal synthesis of calcitriol, which is believed to be the primary cause of SHPT. Failure in managing the serum PTH level may lead to serious clinical consequences including renal osteodystrophy, calcific uremic arteriolopathy, and vascular calcifications that increase morbidity and mortality. SHPT was traditionally managed by intravenous injection of cacitriol. However, hypercalcemia and hyperphosphatemia have been observed as a dose-limiting side effect. In addition to inducing ectopic calcification, hypercalcemia also oversuppresses PTH, leading to adynamic bone disorder. A relatively narrow therapeutic window of calcitriol in effectively reducing PTH levels promotes development of new efficacious vitamin D analogs with decreased calcemic activity.

Treatment of SHPT with calcitriol has correlated to improved survival of dialysis patients. Enhanced survival was also reported by Kovesdy *et al.* [27] in predialysis CKD patients treated with calcitriol for a median duration of 2.1 years. There was also a trend towards reduced dialysis initiation in the calcitriol cohort of the trial enrolled 520 male US veterans with a mean age of 69.8 years. Details of the study are provided in other chapters. A relatively small number of subjects as well as observational nature of this study, however, warrant a larger, randomized trial to assess the effect of calcitriol on cardiovascular and mortality end points [43].

Calcitriol is believed to induce keratinocyte differentiation, inhibit the proliferation of keratinocyte, T-cell and fibroblast, and inhibit the production of some inflammatory mediators, all contributing to the pathogenesis of psoriasis [44]. Though the more precise mechanism of action remains under investigation, calcitriol (Vectical) was approved for the topical treatment of mild-to-moderate plaque psoriasis in adults (18 years and over) on January 23, 2009. In two multicenter, double-blind trials enrolling a total of 839 patients, more than twenty percent of calcitriol-treated patients were classified as having "clear" or "minimal" disease with a $\geq$2-grade change from baseline after applying calcitriol ointment 3 μg/g to affected areas twice daily for 8 weeks. Hypercalcemia was observed more frequently in calcitriol-treated patients than in placebo group. Other common adverse events associated with calcitriol treatment included laboratory test abnormalities, urine abnormalities, hypercalciuria, and pruritus.

Accumulating evidence supports calcitriol's antineoplastic activity in pre-clinical models of prostate cancer and many other tumor types. These antineoplastic effects were observed, however, at exposures of calcitriol substantially above the physiological concentrations. Induction of apoptosis and inhibition of proliferation have been postulated for calcitriol's actions.

Growth inhibition at 50% of LNCaP prostate cancer cells was observed at the clinically achievable concentration of 1 nmol/L in a dose-dependent manner 6 days after exposure to calcitriol. Androgen receptor (AR) and prostate-specific antigen (PSA) protein, however, were also up-regulated at the same concentration. Due to its effect on PSA production, the antineoplastic activity of calcitriol against prostate cancer is more difficult to be evaluated in clinical setting. In a small trial of 8 subjects, no significant change in serum PSA or free PSA was observed 8 days after a single dose of 0.5 μg/kg of calcitriol [45]. Thus, a PSA flare as shown in preclinical settings didnot occur in patients.

A continuous hepatic arterial infusion of calcitriol upto 10 μg/day for 4 weeks observed no side effects including hypercalcemia in a small cohort of patients [46]. The lack of side effects for the hepatic regional administration may allow calcitriol in the treatment of hepatic cancers.

Calcitriol has also been demonstrated to enhance the activity of a variety of chemotherapeutic agents including gemcitabine, the standard care of chemotherapeutic agent to treat pancreatic cancer, *in vitro* and *in vivo,* in multiple tumor models [47]. In a Capan-1 mouse xenograft model, calcitriol in combination with gemcitabine significantly delayed the tumor growth compared to single agent. Promotion of caspase-dependent apoptosis in the combination group may contribute to the increased anti-tumor activity compared to either agent alone. However, there was limited success of calcitriol as a stand-alone intervention in many clinical studies in cancer patients [48].

DOXERCALCIFEROL

Doxercalciferol is a 1α-hydroxy analog of vitamin D_2 and is marketed by Genzyme/Sanofi as the prescription drug Hectorol. Doxercalciferol is indicated for the treatment of SHPT in Stage 3/4 or dialysis CKD patients. Hecterol is available in oral capsules of 0.5 and 2.5 μg, and for intravenous injection in ampoules of 2 and 4 μg. The recommended initial dose of doxercalciferol in dialysis patients is 10μg administered three times weekly at dialysis, and 1 μg administered once daily for non-dialysis patients. However, conclusive data from a head-to-head comparison in the efficacy of intravenous doxercalciferol *vs.* an oral administration are not available [49]. Doxercalciferol is a prodrug and is metabolized to the active hormone $1,25(OH)_2D_2$ in liver by the putative CYP27A1. Bioavailability from a single 5 μg doxercalciferol oral capsule dose was estimated to be normally ~42% of that from a 5 μg intravenous injection. Steady state serum concentrations of $1,25(OH)_2D_2$ were attainable within 8 days, and fluctuated ~2.5-fold from peak to trough when oral doxercalciferol doses were taken every second day, and the terminal half-life was 34 ± 14 h. In several clinical studies, ~74% of pre-dialysis CKD patients treated with Hectorol 0.5 μg capsules achieved a greater than or equal to 30 percent reduction in PTH, which was statistically superior comparing to placebo results. The incidences of hypercalcemia and hyperphosphatemia were similar to placebo therapy, and no episodes of hypercalcemia were observed. Doxercalciferol is recommended as a formulary alternative for patients unresponsive to or intolerant of other vitamin D therapies, but comparative randomized studies to demonstreate a lower incidence of hypercalcemia and/or hyperphosphatemia in relation to other vitamin D therapies are not available. The only comparative trial of doxercalciferol with other vitamin D analog, paricalcitol, was designed for comparing relative dose equivalency, not safety and effectiveness [50]. In a recent randomized, blinded, 3-month trial enrolling vitamin D-deficient CKD stage 3 and 4 patients with elevated PTH values (based on the Kidney Disease Outcomes Quality Initiative gudielines), no significant difference was observed in the efficacy in reduction of PTH levels between cholecalciferol (4000 IU/d x 1 month, then 2000 IU/d; n = 22) and doxercalciferol (1 μg/d; n = 25) [51]. The major adverse effects with the use of doxercalciferol include hypercalcemia and hyperphosphatemia, accompanied by clinical signs of nausea and vomiting, excessive thirst, frequent urination, prerenal azotemia, constipation, abdominal pain, muscle weakness, and muscle and joint aches. Greater dose of oral phosphate binders is typically required in combination to the doxercalciferol therapy.

Doxercalciferol has also been evaluated in patients with advanced hormone-refractory prostate cancer, but further clinical investigation with doxercalciferol alone or in combination with other chemotherapy agents should be conducted for a more conclusive efficacy [52].

PARICALCITOL

Paricalcitol (Zemplar®, Abbott) is a synthetic vitamin D_2 analog. It is available as a sterile, clear, colorless aqueous solution for intravenous injection or in oral capsules. An improved protocol of purifying paricalcitol by crystallization in a mixture of carboxylic acid/hydrocarbon or water has been recently reported [53]. The paricalcitol API (Active Pharmaceutical Ingredient) with greater than 99.7% purity can also be obtained by crystallization from solution in isopropyl acetate following by filtration and vacuum drying [54]. These recently released methods provide simple processes for the purification of crude paricalcitol into API quality material. With this protocol, recovery of paricalcitol was usually greater than 80% and the amount of C-20 epimer was reduced by at least 60%. In addition, paricalcitol with purity over 99.9% appears to have increased storage stability compared to less pure but still pharmaceutically acceptable material. Initially discovered in Deluca's laboratory and later licensed to Abbott Laboratories, paricalcitol mimics the actions of the active D hormone calcitriol. Through binding to VDR, paricalcitol inhibits the secretion of PTH and effectively reduces elevated serum PTH levels. Paricalcitol was approved in the US in 1998 and later in most European nations for the prevention and treatment of SHPT associated with CKD in adult and paediatric (in the US) patients.

The binding affinity of paricalcitol to VDR is 7-fold less that of calcitriol [55]. Paricalcitol inhibits the secretion of PTH at 3- to 10-fold higher dose of calcitriol and in a dose-dependent manner [56]. In uraemic rats, paricalcitol was found to suppress parathyroid hyperplasia and reduce the serum level of PTH [57]. Paricalcitol is also less potent *in vitro* than calcitriol in the stimulation of bone resorption [58]. Paricalcitol is 10-fold less active than calcitriol on raising serum calcium and/or phosphorus levels in animal models.

In well designed clinical trials, paricalcitol was as effective as calcitriol and as well tolerated in terms of the incidence of prolonged hypercalcaemia and/or elevated calcium-phosphorus product. The efficacy of intravenous paricalcitol in the treatment of SHPT has been extensively reviewed by Robinson *et al.* [59]. In several randomized, double-blind, multicenter trials, cohort of adult patients with CKD undergoing haemodialysis were divided into placebo, standard of care controlled, or paricalcitol groups with differing criteria for serum PTH levels. Reduction in mean serum intact PTH (iPTH) levels was observed in a dose-dependent manner over a range of doses (0.04-0.24 μg/kg). Majority of the paricalcitol recipients achieved at least 30% reduction in mean serum iPTH levels after 4 weeks of treatment. In two placebo-controlled trials [60, 61], paricalcitol caused very little change in mean serum phosphorus levels, but induced a small but significant rise (*vs.* baseline) in mean serum calcium levels.

In noncomparative multicenter longer-term studies, up to 59% and 82% reduction in mean iPTH levels, respectively, were achieved after 13 and 16 month therapy with paricalcitol. Resistance often developed after 6-month with calcitriol but a switch to paricalcitol therapy elicited a sustained reduction in serum iPTH levels. The mean serum calcium or phosphorus levels remained largely unchanged during the treatment period. The most serious treatment-related adverse effect was an increased incidence of hypercalcemia and/or hyperphosphatemia in addition to minor adverse events such as nausea, vomiting and oedema. No difference was observed between paricalcitol and calcitriol groups on induction of hypercalcemia or hyperphosphatemia [59-61].

Paricalcitol displayed superior benefit in small cohort of chronic haemodialysis patients compared to calcitriol for the treatment of severe SHPT [62]. In this single centre randomized trial enrolling 25 patients, serum iPTH levels were significantly reduced (P = 0.003) only in the intravenous paricalcitol group but not in the calcitriol group (P = 0.101). On the other hand, serum calcium levels were significantly increased only in the calcitriol group (P = 0.004 *vs.* P = 0.242). Serum phosphorus, alkaline phosphatase and calcium x phosphorus product were not different.

In an attempt to determine the cost effectiveness of paricalcitol *vs.* calcitriol for the treatment of SHPT in CKD patients, Nuijten *et al.* employed a robust Markov model to analyze all data sources of paricalcitol *vs.* calcitriol from published clinical trials and observational studies, official US price/tariff lists and national population statistics. This model showed that the use of paricalcitol is favorable, and leads to an increase in life-years gained (0.47 years) and a gain in number of quality-adjusted life-years (QALYs) (0.43), as well as a cost saving of US$1941/year [63].

Abbott launched in May 2005 an oral formulation of Zemplar in capsule that is indicated for the prevention and treatment of SHPT associated with Stage 3 and 4 CKD before the need for dialysis or transplantation. The safety and efficacy of Zemplar Capsules were evaluated in three, 24-week, double blind, placebo-controlled, randomized, multicenter, Phase 3 clinical studies in CKD Stage 3 and 4 patients. The results showed that 91% of Zemplar treated patients *vs.* 13% of the placebo (p <0.001) achieved the primary efficacy endpoint of at least two consecutive ≥30% reduction in PTH from baseline. The proportion of Zemplar Capsules treated patients achieving two consecutive ≥30% reduction in PTH was similar between the daily and the three times a week regimens (daily: 30/33, 91%; three times a week: 62/68, 91%). No increase in incidences of hypercalcemia (defined as two consecutive serum calcium values >10.5 mg/dL), hyperphosphatemia and elevated Ca x P product were observed in Zemplar Capsules treated patients as compared to placebo.

In a recent trial published by Lund *et al.* [64], the intestinal Ca^{2+} absorption in hemodialysis patients treated with calcitriol *vs.* paricalcitol at a dose ratio 1:3 was evaluated. A total of 22 patients aged ≥20 years on maintenance hemodialysis for more than 2 months (including 2 month) with iPTH levels at >200 pg/ml were enrolled in the single-center, double-blind, active-controlled, randomized, crossover trial. It was found that the paricalcitol-treated patients absorbed approximately 14% less Ca^{2+} compared with calcitriol-treated patients with similar effects on PTH. Overall Ca^{2+} absorption was relatively low in this patient cohort, indicating that regulation of Ca^{2+} absorption may be dysfunctional. There were no significant differences in serum PTH, Ca^{2+}, phosphorus (P), or Ca x P.

Due to its potential in reducing proteinuria, paricalcitol was evaluated for the treatment of proteinuric renal diseases [65]. Sixty one patients of proteinuric CKD with estimated glomerular filtration rate (eGFR) at 15 to 90 mL/min/1.73 m^2 and protein excretion greater than 400 mg/24 h were enrolled into a double-blind randomized clinical study. Paricalcitol was administered orally at 1 µg/d *vs.* placebo for 6 month. Serum iPTH, calcium, phosphorus, creatinine, and urine spot protein and creatinine were measured every 4 weeks. Mean urinary protein-creatinine ratios between the baseline measurement and the last study evaluation were determined to be 2.6 and 2.8 g/g in the placebo and paricalcitol groups, respectively. At final evaluation, mean ratios were 2.7 and 2.3, respectively. Changes in protein excretion from baseline to last evaluation were +2.9% for controls and -17.6% for the paricalcitol group (P = 0.04). A significant reduction in protein excretion in patients with proteinuric renal disease was observed for paricalcitol.

Paricalcitol also appears to be effective in reducing albuminuria in patients with Type II diabetes. In a multinational, double-blind clinical trial, 283 Type II diabetic patients receiving the standard of care including RAAS (renin-angiotensin-aldosterone system) inhibitors were divided into placebo (n = 93), 1 µg/day (n = 93) or 2 µg/day (n = 95) of oral paricalcitol cohorts. The combined paricalcitol groups observed a -16% (from 62 to 51 mg/mmol) change in geometric mean urinary albumin/creatinine ratio (UACR) following 24 weeks of treatment, while the change in UACR was -3% (from 61 to 60 mg/mmol) for the placebo. Patients on 2 µg paricalcitol showed an early, sustained reduction in UACR, ranging from -18% to -28% (p = 0.014 *vs.* placebo). However, no statistically significant difference for adverse events was observed among these groups [66].

Paricalcitol has also been evaluated as a potential agent in treating myelodysplastic syndrome (MDS) primarily due to the anti-proliferative effect and induction of differentiation of the vitamin D hormone. However, all clinical studies, either alone or in combination with other chemical agents including inhibitors of the mitochondrial enzyme CYP24A1, have not generated conclusive data although hypercalcemia was rarely detected [67, 68]. The preliminary benefit of paricalcitol on improving endothelial function, blood pressure, albuminuria, and inflammation has been observed in CKD patients [69]. In a mouse unilateral ureteral obstruction (UUO) model of nephropathy, paricalcitol displayed synergistic effects with a RAAS inhibitor, Trandolapril, in reducing renal fibrosis [70]. In addition, a number of animal studies demonstrated that paricalcitol may have the potential to serve as an adjuvant agent for the treatment of disease conditions such as rheumatoid arthritis [71] and atherosclerosis [72].

CALCIPOTRIOL

Calcipotriol, also called calcipotriene or MC-903, is probably one of the best known synthetic derivatives of vitamin D. Available as cream, ointment and scalp solution (50 µg/mL), calcipotriol is indicated as the first-line treatment for plaque psoriasis under the trade name of Dovonex or Daivonex. Improvement is usually observed following two weeks of topical application. Calcipotriol has shown efficacy in clinical trials with minimal hypercalcemia. The most common adverse effect is skin irritation at the site of application. Calcipotriol is also available in combination with the synthetic glucocorticoid betamethasone under the trade name Taclonex, Dovobet or Daivobet. When applied once daily for psoriasis, the combined formulation of calcipotriol and betamethasone dipropionate (the TCF gel) is considered to be the most efficacious treatment for plaque psoriasis among the topical therapies evaluated in terms of PASI (Psoriasis Area and Severity Index) score [73, 74]. A meta-analysis has also suggested that the TCF gel has significant benefits over other topical therapies in the routine management of patients with moderate-severe scalp psoriasis [75]. The TCF gel is convenient, with a faster speed of onset and greater efficacy than its individual active ingredient. Most patients observed obvious efficacy with absent or very mild disease following 2 weeks of topical application and the percentage of responding patients increases to ~70% after 8 weeks of therapy. The combination formulation is well tolerated with a safety profile similar to betamethasone dipropionate alone and significantly fewer cutaneous adverse events as compared to calcipotriene [76].

Greater efficacy with regard to the reduction in PASI was also observed for the combined ointment formulation of calcipotriol and corticosteroid than by using either compound alone in a multicenter, prospective, randomized, and double-blind clinical trial [77]. In this international clinical trial, one of the four patient cohorts was treated with the two-in-one formulation once daily, while the other three groups were treated with the vehicle ointment, calcipotriol ointment, or the corticosteroid formulation twice daily for 4 weeks in psoriasis vulgaris amendable for topical treatments. Fewer adverse events were observed in the combined formulation group than in both the calcipotriol group and the vehicle group. When compared to vehicle ointment or calcipotriol ointment alone, the combined regiments were shown to be clearly more efficacious.

In a randomized, investigator blinded trial enrolled 458 patients with at least moderate-severe psoriasis vulgaris, the two-compound formulation (calcipotriol plus betamethasone dipropionate gel) also compared favorably relative to calcipotriol ointment in both efficacy and safety. This 8-week trial was investigator blinded, and the treatment success was defined as patients with a 'clear' or 'almost clear' at Week 8. The proportion of patients who were 'clear or almost clear' was significantly higher in the two-compound formulation group (39.9%) compared with 17.9% in the calcipotriol group (p <0.001). Less proportion of patients with at least one adverse drug reaction was observed in the 2-compound gel group [78].

Calcipotriol may be beneficial to other skin disorders including morphoea, palmoplantar pustulosis, ichthyosis, keratoderma, and Grover's disease [79]. No significant efficacy was observed, however, for topical application of calcipotriol to reduce hypertrophic scar formation in a randomized, double-blind, placebo-controlled trial [80]. Dovonex is not recommended for use on the face, where the skin is particularly sensitive.

Since the effectiveness of vitamin D analogs in treating psoriasis was first discovered accidentally in an osteoporosis clinical study in 1985, psoriasis remains to be one of the major research areas in the vitamin D field. Calcipotriol works primarily by slowing the rate at which psoriatic skin cells multiply, and by making newly-formed skin cells differentiate into their proper forms. However, the precise mechanism of action in remitting psoriasis is not well-understood yet. Although calcipotriol is only 1% as active as calcitriol in regulating calcium metabolism, calcipotriol has been shown to have comparable affinity as calcitriol to VDR in human epidermal keratinocytes, dermal fibrinoblasts and lymphocytes. At appropriate concentrations, calcipotriol causes a decrease in the proliferation and an increase in the morphologic and biochemical differentiation of keratinocytes, hence regulating their proliferation and differentiation. Calcipotriol helps to control psoriasis by slowing down the production of new skin cells. Although many treatment options are available to control symptoms and minimize the impact of psoriasis on daily activities, effective psoriasis treatment remains a challenge. Currently, calcipotriol is one of the most popular topical treatments for this condition.

SEOCALCITOL

Seocalcitol, also called EB1089, is one of the vitamin D side chain analogs that displays up to two logs of higher potency than calcitriol for cell differentiation *in vitro* with a reduced calcaemic activity *in vivo*. In preclinical models, seocalcitol significantly inhibited the growth of N-methyl-nitrosourea (NMU)-induced rat mammary tumor with a significant increase in serum and urinary calcium levels [81]. Using the NMU-induced tumor model with consideration of a balance between obtaining maximal efficacy and an acceptable safety profile, an optimal dosing regimen is believed to be close to 1 µg/kg daily for 4 weeks or the same total dose of seocalcitol administered every 10th day (8 µg/kg 3 times). This relatively low calcaemic activity observed in animals was translated into human clinical results early on. Furthermore, seocalcitol has been shown to induce regression of tumors, especially in hepatocellular carcinoma where complete remission has been obtained [82]. Interaction with the estrogen pathway and down-regulation of the expression of progesterone receptor by seocalcitol are believed to be the primary mode of action [83].

Seocalcitol, in a mouse MCF-7 breast tumor xenograft model, enhanced the sensitivity of the breast tumor cells to both adriamycin and ionizing radiation, in part through the promotion of apoptotic cell death [84, 85]. Final tumor volumes in animals irradiated after the seocalcitol treatment for 8 days were 50% lower than in the group that received radiation alone. This findingcorrelated to an increased number of non-proliferative cells and apoptotic cells in tumors irradiated after seocalcitol [86]. Inoperable cancer of the exocrine pancreas responds poorly to most conventional anti-cancer agents. Seocalcitol can inhibit growth, induce differentiation and apoptosis *in vitro*, and can also inhibit growth of pancreatic cancer xenografts *in vivo* [87].

Seocalcitol also induces apoptosis of human ovarian cancer cells *in vitro* and in nude mice. It significantly suppressed the growth of OVCAR3 xenografts in nude mice at a non-hypercalcemic dose [88]. Both decreased cell proliferation and increased cell death are believed to contribute to the antitumor activity.

Unfortunately, the performance of seocalcitol in clinical settings has not been consistent. In a phase II study enrolling 56 patients with inoperable hepatocellular carcinoma (HCC), 2 out of 33 patients achieved complete response, 12 remained stable and 19 continued to progress following the seocalcitol treatment for one year [89]. Most patients tolerated a daily dose of 10 μg of seocalcitol with hypercalcemia and related symptoms as the most frequent toxicity. Cessation of treatment or administration of a lower dose (1 μg/kg twice weekly) reversed hypercalcemia, hypercalciuria and weight loss induced by high dose seocalcitol. This was the first study of seocalcitol showing efficacy in patients with an advanced bulky, solid tumor. Seocalcitol may have an effect in the treatment of HCC, especially in an early disease stage when a prolonged treatment can be instituted. The survival benefit with or without tumor response should be determined in controlled studies. Higher response rate may be achieved, however, by selecting patients whose tumor expresses the VDR, though information on patient's VDR status is difficult to obtain in the clinical setting. In another phase II study enrolling 36 patients with advanced pancreatic cancer, only 14 of them completed 8 weeks of the seocalcitol treatment. Twenty patients deteriorated clinically and were withdrawn from the study prior to completing the treatment. Thus, no objective tumor responses were observed in these 14 patients at doses up to 30μg/day, although the treatment seemed relatively safe [90]. Development of seocalcitol as single agent for the cancer indication was discontinued.

TACALCITOL

Tacalcitol (Teijin Ltd) is a 1α, 24(R)-dihydroxy analog of vitamin D_3 and structurally similar to calcipotriol where isopropyl is replaced with a cyclopropyl group. Tacalcitol, in ointment form at a concentration of 4 μg/g, is indicated for mild and/or moderate psoriasis (with <20% of the surface of the skin affected) under several names including Curatodem and Bonalfa.

Though exact molecular mechanism is not fully known, evidence has indicated that tacalcitol can influence the principle pathogenetic factors of psoriasis such as inducing keratinocyte differentiation, performing an anti-proliferative action and also modulating the inflammatory response [91]. Tacalcitol binds to the keratinocyte VDR to the same extent as the natural hormone calcitriol. Tacalcitol inhibits the expression of mRNA for the c-fos and c-myc genes that are important for cellular proliferation, as well as expression of cytokeratin 16 and involucrin, which are absent in normal skin but overexpressed in psoriatic lesions.

Treatment of mild/moderate psoriasis with tacalcitol ointment induces a rapid improvement or complete resolution of psoriatic lesion. An improvement can normally be noticed within 2 to 4 weeks following the treatment. The beneficial effect continues with multiple applications and may last even after treatment has stopped. Efficacy of tacalcitol as the first-line monotherapy in the treatment of psoriasis has been extensively reviewed [92, 93]. Its efficacy was found to be comparable to that of topical corticosteroids and also calcipotriol, with a lower percentage of relapses and side effects and greater cosmetic acceptability [92]. Unlike other standard therapies, this product does not have odor and does not stain clothing. Synergistic effect was also observed for tacalcitol ointment in combination with narrow band UVB phototherapy with reduced phototoxic side effects [94]. The common side effects of tacalcitol include temporary irritation of the skin or allergic reactions.

Other than psoriasis, tacalcitol in combination with phototherapy has also demonstrated efficacy for the treatment of vitiligo in patients who have not responded to traditional therapies [95, 96]. In a small clinical trial enrolling 15 patients, 40% reported a clinical response that varied from good to excellent following sequential exposure to solar radiation for 30 minutes and topical application of tacalcitol. The efficacy of tacalcitol in combination with 308-nm monochromatic excimer light (MEL) therapy has also been evaluated in treatment of vitiligo *vs.* MEL 308-nm therapy alone. In the single-blind, open-label study, 32 vitiligo patients were randomly applied with either topical tacalcitol cream or vehicle. Each lesion was treated weekly with the 308-nm MEL for a total of 12 sessions. The treatment with tacalcitol and MEL resulted in higher percentages for excellent repigmentation (25.7%) compared with vehicle and MEL (5.7%) (P <0.05). Percentages of total response were 71.4% and 60%, respectively (P >0.05). The results demonstrate that concurrent topical tacalcitol potentiates the efficacy of the 308-nm MEL in the treatment of vitiligo, and that this combination achieves earlier pigmentation with a lower total dosage [97]. These clinical observations, however, are different from that found in a more recent and relatively larger clinical trial. A single-center, randomized, and double-blind clinical regimen enrolling 80 patients with nonsegmental vitiligo was conducted in an effort to investigate the efficacy and safety of tacalcitol ointment plus sunlight exposure. Efficacy was assessed by quantification of the lesional repigmentation area at the end of the study compared with the baseline. After daily exposures to sunlight for 30 minutes, tacalcitol (n = 40) or matching placebo ointment (n = 40) was applied once a day at night continuously for 4 months. Despite of lack of adverse events, the combination of tacalcitol with heliotherapy displayed no additional advantages compared with heliotherapy alone in [98]. Individual cases have also been reported for tacalcitol to be effective in treating verruciform epidermodysplasia [99] and Grover's disease [100].

MAXACALCITOL

Maxacalcitol (OCT) is an 22-oxa-derivative of $1\alpha,25$-dihydroxyvitamin D_3 that is currently indicated for SHPT and psoriasis under brand name Oxarol. Synthesized from 1α-hydroxydehydroepiandrosterone at industrial scale [101], maxacalcitol displaya approximately 10 times greater potentcy at suppressing proliferation and inducing differentiation of epidermal keratinocytes *in vitro* than calcipotriol and tacalcitol. It is the first vitamin D analog that exerts a selective action on the parathyroid gland. Maxacalcitol has a very short half–life in blood circulation with a persistent accumulation in the parathyroid gland, thus eliciting selective suppression of PTH. The increased selectivity of maxacalcitol in suppressing PTH in animal CKD models has been demonstrated in several laboratories [102]. Observations in clinical settings agreed well with the preclinical findings. In two randomized clinical trials enrolling 124 and 101 hemodialysis patients, treatment with maxacalcitol for one year achieved the target PTH reduction in 64 (52%) and 44 (44%) patients, respectively. Higher dose appeared to correlate to an increased percentage of patients who achieved 30% PTH reduction, and exhibited increased serum calcium and phosphate levels, and elevated calcium x phosphate product, albeit within the normal ranges.

The improved selectivity of maxacalcitol for PTH observed in preclinical models, however, was not confirmed in a head-to-head comparison of intravenous maxacalcitol (thrice weekly) with oral calcitriol in a small trial of 23 patients over 24 weeks. At doses for minimized hypercalcemia, both trial arms demonstrated similar 35% reduction in PTH levels, similar increases in serum calcium levels, and no significant difference in episodes of elevated Ca xP product. In an attempt to minimize the impact from different routes of administration, a larger randomized prospective multicenter trial to compare intravenous maxacalcitol (44 patients) and intravenous calcitriol (47 patients) in chronic haemeodialysis patients was conducted. Again, no statistical advantage in favor of maxacalcitol was observed [103]. Although caution should be paid to the onset of hypercalcemia and oversuppression of PTH, maxacalcitol is one of the effective tools for the treatment of SHPT.

For patients with advanced SHPT (A-SHPT) resistant to conventional medical treatment, ultrasound-guided direct injection of maxacalcitol into the hyperplastic parathyroid gland (PTG) was recommended [104]. The initial dose was set at 10 μg, but this was adjusted later according to serum calcium and iPTH levels that were measured every 4 weeks. Under the guideline of the Japanese Society for Parathyroid Intervention, maxacalcitol was directly injected into hyperplastic PTG daily for 6 days followed by intravenous administration at the end of each hemodialysis. Serum iPTH levels were found to decrease significantly and maintained for at least 12 weeks. Suppression of PTH synthesis and secretion, upregulation of both VDR and calcium-sensing receptor (CaSR), and induction of parathyroid cell (PTC) apoptosis by maxacalcitol appeared to be responsible for its efficacy.

Since the market launch of "maxacalcitol ointment" in October 2001, maxacalcitol has been widely used in Japan in patients with keratosis including psoriasis vulgaris. In a phase II double-blind, randomized trial, 144 patients with mild to moderate chronic plaque psoriasis were treated once-daily with topical maxacalcitol ointment at a variety of concentration of 6, 12.5, 25 and 50 µg/g for 8 weeks. Psoriasis severity index (PSI) based on sum of scores for erythema, scaling and induration together with investigators' overall assessment were used as primary parameters to assess efficacy. While all concentrations of maxacalcitol remarkably improved the symptoms, the 25 µg/g ointment displayed the greatest effect which compared favorably with calcipotriol ointment 50 µg/g once daily. Improvement continued throughout the study period, with no plateau at week 8 [105]. Recently a more cosmetically friendly lotion formulation was developed for the treatment of psoriatic lesions on the face and scalp, which demonstrated a similar cutaneous bioavailability compared to the maxacalcitol ointment [106].

For patients with moderate psoriasis vulgaris whose disease activity had been unchanged or exacerbated with topical maxacalcitol treatment, a supplementary cyclosporin microemulsion preconcentrate (CyA MEPC) has been recommended [107]. In a small 15-patient trial, each patient took a supplementary CyA MEPC administration, 2.5 mg/kg per day, in addition to maxacalcitol ointment therapy. When the Psoriasis Area and Severity Index (PASI) score revealed over a 75% decrease against the initial value, the administration of CyA MEPC was tapered off, and a topical application of maxacalcitol ointment was continued for the maintenance phase. All patients obtained improvement within 12 weeks.

Topical maxacalcitol is also effective against viral warts, a refractory but common benign tumors caused by human papilloma viruses. Application of maxacalcitol ointment (25 µg/g) three times a day for 2 weeks to 6 months completely cleared the symptom of all 17 patients [108].

Maxacalcitol ointment also appeared to be effective in the treatment of infantile acropustulosis (IA), pruritic vesiculo-pustular eruption on palms and soles [109]. New eruptions decreased, and all eruptions disappeared completely following twice a day application of maxacalcitol ointment (25 µg/g) for one week. Application of maxacalcitol every 3 - 4 days was continued and the interval between occurrences gradually increased. The approximate applied dose of maxacalcitol was at a maximum of 10g/month. Inhibition of the expression of cytokines such as interleukin (IL)-1α, IL-6 and IL-8 from keratinocytes is proposed to be responsible for its efficacy. Though calcium levels were not monitored, but no clinical symptoms of hypercalcaemia were observed.

Based on reviewing and analyzing the literature reports from 1980 to 2008, de Jager and co-workers have assessed the efficacy and safety of current treatments for childhood psoriasis and recommended a general guideline [110]. Calcipotriene, or in combination with corticosteroids if needed, was recommended for mild or moderate childhood psoriasis. In case of treatment-resistant flexural and/or facial psoriasis, tacrolimus 0.1% can be added to the treatment regimen. If this treatment regimen fails, treatment with dithranol is then recommended. Only in case of lack of efficacy of these modalities, treatment with NB-UVB can be considered in adolescents, but only for a short duration.

FALECALCITRIOL

Falecalcitriol is an analog of 1α,25-dihydroxyvitamin D_3 in which the hydrogens on both Carbon 26 and 27 have been completely substituted with fluorine atoms. Falecalcitriol displays 10 to 100-fold higher potency than calcitriol *in vitro* depending on the target organs [111]. Primarily due to a strong electron-withdrawing effect of the fluorine substituents, falecalcitriol displays a longer half-life than calcitriol and can be converted to a more stable 23-hydroxylated metabolite *in vivo*. The C-23S hydroxylated metabolite exhibits higher activities in bone, parathyroid cells, and keratinocytes when compared with calcitriol. Falecalcitriol demonstrates clinical effects for the treatment of diseases such as SHPT in CKD, rickets, and osteomalacia at doses lower than those required for calcitriol. Falecalcitriol is orally active, and believed to offer a safer and more effective way of controlling SHPT without the intravenous route.

In an initial clinical study by Nishizawa *et al.*, 43 patients with CKD were given oral falecalcitriol daily starting at a dose of 0.05 µg/day. This dose was increased every two weeks until hypercalcemia appeared. At the end of the 12-week clinical regimen, the mean reduction in serum level of serum iPTH was 25% with minimal change in serum calcium [112].

To compare the clinical effects of oral falecalcitriol treatment with those of intravenous calcitriol, 21 patients with moderate to severe SHPT were included in a random 2 x 2 crossover 12-week trial. A similar decrease in iPTH and whole PTH (wPTH) levels was observed in both treatment groups. Serum levels of Ca^{2+}, P, and Ca x P product at the end of each treatment appeared to be similar. This study showed that both oral falecalcitriol treatment and intravenous calcitriol administration were effective for PTH suppression, and also exhibited similar effects on Ca^{2+} and P metabolism in hemodialysis patients with moderate to severe SHPT, but no advantage was observed for falecalcitriol during this study [113]. Another comparative study of falecarcitriol with alfacalcidol showed its specific action on PTH suppression and better improvement of bone metabolism markers in SHPT patients [114].

Falecalcitriol appeared to be effective in CKD patients on continuous ambulatory peritoneal dialysis (CAPD) who failed conventional vitamin D therapy [115]. Both intact and whole PTH levels of a 55 year old Japanese man with end-stage renal disease continued to rise following the treatment with alfacalcidol up to a dose of 0.75 µg/day, in combination with $CaCO_3$ (1.5 g/day). Switching to falecalcitriol at 0.3 µg/day decreased both iPTH and wPTH levels more than 4-fold, without any drug-related adverse reactions. However, caution should be paid to patients who receive falecalcitriol together with phosphate binder such as $CaCO_3$ to avoid hypercalcemia due to increased intestinal absorption of calcium.

ELDECALCITOL

Developed by Chugai, eldecalcitol (ED-71) is a 3-hydroxypropoxy analog at 2β-position of 1α,25-dihydroxyvitamin D_3, and binds to the VDR with approximately a third of the affinity of 1α,25(OH)$_2$D$_3$. Primarily due to a higher affinity for the DBP, eldecalcitol appears to have a longer half-life in circulation than calcitriol does, and seems to have stronger effecte in bone [116, 117]. In ovariectomized rats, eldecalcitol increased lumbar vertebral bone mass and bone strength by inhibiting bone resorption and maintaining bone formation without causing hypercalcemia [118]. Clinical studies have shown that treatment with eldecalcitol effectively and safely increased lumbar and hip bone mineral density (BMD) in osteoporotic patients, which represents a promising new therapy for osteoporosis. For example, in a randomized, double-blind, placebo-controlled trial enrolling 219 osteoporotic patients, 0.50, 0.75 or 1.00 µg/day eldecalcitol or vehicle were given for 12 months, in addition to 200 or 400 IU/day vitamin D_3. A dose-dependent increase in lumbar and hip BMD was observed in the eldecalcitol cohort. In addition, bone formation and resorption markers decreased by ~20% after 12 months of treatment. Although transient hypercalcemia arose in 7% (0.50 µg), 5% (0.75 µg) and 23% (1.00 µg) of patients treated with eldecalcitol, none developed sustained hypercalcemia [119]. These findings compared favorably to the data obtained with alfacalcidol in term of an increase in BMD with similar effects on serum and urinary calcium. A 0.75 µg/day dose was recommended to be a "safe, well-tolerated and effective dose in increasing both lumbar and femoral BMD". A post-hoc analysis was also conducted to evaluate the impact of 25(OH)D levels on the efficacy of eldecalcitol. It was found that lumbar BMD following 12-month treatment with 0.5, 0.75 and 1.0 µg/day eldecalcitol increased similarly in both lower (<25 ng/mL) and upper tertile (>29 ng/mL) groups of serum 25(OH)D, suggesting that eldecalcitol may exert its effect as a unique VDR ligand with stronger effect on bone compared to the natural ligand, 1,25(OH)$_2$D$_3$ [120]. Several of these prospective, randomized, and double-blind Phase III studies to compare the effect of eldecalcitol with that of alfacalcidol in osteoporotic patients have been completed. A new drug application for osteoporosis has been submitted in 2009.

ELOCALCITOL

Initially developed by Roche Bioscience and later licensed to BioXell, elocalcitol (BXL-628 or Ro-26-9228) is another analog of calcitriol that possesses much of the desired properties of the natural hormone, but is devoid of a hypercalcemic effect. Elocalcitol is being developed for benign prostatic hyperplasia (BPH) and overactive bladder (OAB).

Despite less active than calcitriol, elocalcitol displays a wider therapeutic window than calcitriol in a number of preclinical disease models. Elocalcitol demonstrated a bone-protecting effect in an ovariectomy-induced osteoporosis rat model at an oral dose of 3 μg/kg/day and above, and did not cause hypercalcemia at the maximum tested dose of 14 μg/kg/day [121]. As a comparison, calcitriol induced hypercalcemia at 0.2 μg/kg/day, a dose required for bone protection. Unlike calcitriol, elocalcitol upregulated osteoblast-specific genes and bone growth factors without affecting genes in the duodenum. Both calcitriol and elocalcitol promote the expression of osteopontin and osteocalcin genes with ED_{50} values of 0.8 - 5.5 nM in human osteoblast-like ROS 17/2.8 and hFOB cells and osteosarcoma MG-63 cells. Their activities in human Caco-2 cells, however, are different that calcitriol is 60-fold more potent in inducing osteocalcin gene expression with an ED_{50} of 2 nM. Calcitriol also appears to be more active in inducing the expression of calbindin D9K mRNA with an ED_{50} of 5-8 nM, 20-fold more potent than elocalcitol. Elocalcitol inhibits the proliferation of benign prostatic hyperplasia (BPH) cells more potently than finasteride, a 5α-reductase inhibitor.

In rat BPH models, elocalcitol significantly decreased prostate growth at an oral dose of 10-300 μg/kg in both intact and castrated rats supplemented with testosterone. In a female rat model of bladder outlet obstruction, bladder wall hypertrophy was induced to an equal extent in rats treated with either elocalcitol or vehicle. However, in the elocalcitol-treated rats contractile function was maintained, whereas function decreased in the vehicle-treated animals. *Ex vivo* analysis of bladder muscle strips showed that the bladder muscle of elocalcitol-treated rats remained responsive to nerve stimulation, while reduced contractile responses were observed for the bladder muscle of vehicle-treated rats [122].

Elocalcitol has been evaluated clinically for osteoporosis in a double-blind, randomized study enrolling 101 postmenopausal osteoporotic women. All subjects received 1.2 g/day calcium and 400 IU vitamin D/day together with elocalcitol (150 μg/day P.O.) or placebo for 90 days. Significant efficacy with an increase in whole-body BMD and a decrease in markers of bone formation and resorption was observed for the treatment group without causing hypocalcaemia. In a milti-center, double-blind, randomized, placebo-controlled Phase IIa clinical trial, the efficacy and safety of elocalcitol was assessed for the treatment of BPH. One hundred and nineteen eligible patients of diagnosed non-malignant BPH with prostate volume of ≥40 mL were enrolled into the study. Following a 12-week study, the elocalcitol treatment cohort demonstrated statistically positive results in terms of reduction of prostate volume (7.2%) *vs.* placebo (p <0.0001), responded rate (92 *vs.* 48% in elocalcitol-treated *vs.* placebo), and high safety/tolerability [123].

A follow-on phase IIb trial for the same indication was then conducted, which exhibited a similar spectrum of activities in a larger 514 patients group. The primary endpoint was met with a high degree of statistical significance, with elocalcitol effectively arresting prostate growth. Elocalcitol also showed relevant effects on the symptomatic parameters such as urgency, frequency and nocturia, as well as on the urodynamic parameter maximum urinary flow rate (Qmax). However, phase IIb trial data from patients with overactive bladder (OAB) were less promising with elocalcitol failing to meet the primary endpoint. Despite of the novel mechanism of action, efficacy profile and improved tolerability of elocalcitol over existing classes of drugs, BioXell decided in April 2009 to terminate all further clinical development of elocalcitol, including an uncompleted phase IIa trial in patients with male infertility [124]. Beforehand, the company also communicated its decision to suspend the Phase II trial of elocalcitol in male infertility. All research activities with regards to the company's vitamin D analogs have been terminated [125].

CTA018

Discovered at Prof. Posner's laboratory at The Johns Hopkins University, CTA018 Injection contains a conceptually novel sulfone analog of the hormone 1α,25-dihydroxyvitamin D_3. They substituted the side chain of the vitamin D hormone with a tert-butyl sulfone in which the sulfone oxygen mimics the Lewis basic hydroxyl group on the steroid side chain. An established 16, 23-diene was also incorporated into the molecule for a decreased episodic calcemic function [126]. This designed hybrid exhibits a dual mechanism of action that combines the vitamin D hormone function in activating VDR with CYP24A1 inhibition. As discussed earlier and also in other chapters, expression of CYP24A1 is elevated as the intracellular levels of the vitamin D hormone rise to limit exposure, thereby preventing toxicity. Prolonged vitamin D analog therapy therefore induces CYP24A1 expression to levels that may limit effectiveness of therapy. Deletion of CYP24A1 in mice resulted in decreased clearance of 1α,25-dihydroxyvitamin D_3, leading to increased vitamin D hypersensitivity and soft tissue calcification. Like traditional therapies, CTA018 activates the vitamin D signaling pathway by binding to VDR. Unlike traditional therapies, CTA018 also reduces the catabolism of vitamin D hormones by binding to and thereby blocking CYP24A1.

In preclinical models, CTA018 has demonstrated advantages over two marketed vitamin D hormone replacement therapies, calcitriol and paricalcitol, the latter currently being the most widely used therapy for SHPT in the United States. CTA018 appeared to be 10-fold more potent than calcitriol in activating VDR-mediated gene transcription although its binding affinity for VDR is 15-fold lower. CTA018 is over 10 times more effective in inhibiting CYP24A1 than ketoconazole, one of the most potent non-selective CYP24A1 inhibitors. So, it is highly possible that the discrepancy in VDR binding affinity *vs.* gene transcriptional activity is related to its effect on CYP24A1 [127]. CTA018 was found to have consistent effectiveness in lowering PTH throughout a 4-week treatment period, while paricalcitol became progressively less effective. In addition, CTA018 exhibited a reduced activity and half-life in human enterocytes (intestinal cells), suggesting a wider therapeutic window in inducing episodic hypercalcemia and hyperphosphatemia. The novel dual mechanism of action demonstrated by CTA018 may elicit a desired therapeutic response while reducing clinically acquired resistance to vitamin D hormone therapy caused by CYP24A1. CTA018 Injection may provide a safer and more effective therapeutic option for managing advanced SHPT. However, a word of caution is noted that CTA018 may be solely metabolized by CYP3A, leading to potential drug-drug interaction in patients. CTA018 Injection is under development by Cytochroma for the treatment of SHPT in Stage 5 CKD patients. In an open label, placebo-controlled, and randomized Phase I clinical trial enrolling 20 healthy volunteers, CTA018 Injection was well tolerated and produced clinically meaningful reductions in blood levels of PTH after less than two weeks of administration. No clinically relevant elevations in serum calcium or phosphorus were observed. CTA018 Injection is in Phase II clinical development for the treatment of SHPT in CKD patients undergoing dialysis [128].

2MD

2MD is an unique class of A-ring analog of $1\alpha,25$-dihydroxyvitamin D_3 with transposition of C-19 exocyclic methylene group to C-2 position. Discovered at DeLuca's laboratory at University of Wisconsin [129], 2MD demonstrated two distinctive modes of action, showing activity on both bone resorption and new bone formation [130, 131]. Like traditional vitamin D hormonal analogs, 2MD displays a slightly weaker binding affinity to VDR compared to that of calcitriol, but induces differentiation of HL-60 cells with a similar ED_{50}. Unlike other vitamin D analogs, 2MD also acts as a bone anabolic agent in an ovariectomized rat model, stimulating new bone formation [132]. In a randomized, double-blind, placebo-controlled Phase II trial of osteopenic women, the effect of daily oral treatment with 2MD on BMD, serum markers of bone turnover, and safety was assessed over 1 year. All patients were randomly assigned to three treatment groups: placebo (n = 50), 220 ng of 2MD (n = 54), and 440 ng of 2MD (n = 53). In general, 2MD was well tolerated. Although 2MD caused a significant increase in serum carboxy-terminal collagen cross-links (CTX) and osteocalcin (markers of bone formation), it did not significantly increase BMD [133]. There also observed no statistical changes in bone mineral content or area at week 26 or 52 after a post-hoc analysis. There was a dose-dependent decrease of iPTH at week 26 relative to baseline levels which correlates to biochemical evidence of increased bone turnover.

2MD's lack of efficacy in increasing BMD in osteopenic postmenopausal women is in stark contrast to its effect in the OVX rat, where dramatic increases in BMD were observed. The Wisconsin researchers speculated that the discrepancy could be due to the differences in bone metabolism in rats and humans, and suggested a cautious use of the OVX rat model when developing novel osteoporosis therapies.

CONCLUSION

Selective VDR activators constitute a family of promising vitamin D analogs that regulate multiple aspects of VDR functions. Most of the successful efforts have been achieved in identifying analogs for the treatment of osteoporosis, psoriasis and SHPT in CKD, but research in seeking even more effective analogs for these indications continues. While many analogs show significantly wider therapeutic windows *in vitro* and in pre-clinical animal models, separation of the desired activities such as improved potency without calcemic response become less significant under clinical settings. The numerous crystal structures of VDR reveal the adaptability of the vitamin D ligand along with the potential flexibility of the protein. The vitamin D analogs with differences in biological activities do not exhibit significant change in the binding mode in the X-ray structure of VDR. Challenges therefore remain in structurally designing novel analogs with specific physiological functions. While numerous observational clinical studies demonstrate the efficacy of vitamin D analogs in chemoprevention and chemotherapy, randomized trails are essential and efforts in combination therapy also need to be made. In addition, basic research need to continue to further elucidate the mechanisms by which vitamin D and its analogs act at the cellular and molecular level, and also to identify additional downstream targets in the VDR signaling pathway.

REFERENCES

[1] For recent reviews: see: (a) Mason RS. Vitamin D: a hormone for all seasons. Climacteric 2011; 14(2): 197-203; (b) Cunningham J, Zehnder D. New Vitamin D analogs and changing therapeutic paradigms. Kidney Int 2011; 79(7): 702-707; (c) Borges MC, Martini LA, Rogero MM. Current perspectives on vitamin D, immune system, and chronic diseases. Nutrition 2011; 27(4): 399-404; (d) Tremezaygues L, Reichrath J. From the bench to emerging new clinical concepts: Our present understanding of the importance of the vitamin D endocrine system (VDES) for skin cancer. Dermato-Endocrinology 2011; 3(1): 11-17; (e) Li YC. Podocytes as target of vitamin D. Curr Diabetes Rev 2011; 7(1): 35-40.

[2] Meng H, Chen G, Zhang X, Wang Z, Thomas DG, Giordano TJ, Beer TG, Wang MM. Stromal LRP1 in lung adenocarcinoma predicts clinical outcome. Clin Cancer Res 2011; DOI: 10.1158/1078-0432.ccr-10-2385.

[3] For extensive reviews, see: (a) Agoston ES, Hatcher MA, Kensler TW, Posner GH. Vitamin D analogs as anti-carcinogenic agents. Anti-Cancer Agents Med Chem 2006; 6(1): 53-71; (b) Saito N, Honzawa S, Kittaka A. Recent results on A-ring modification of 1α,25-dihydroxyvitamin D_3: design and synthesis of VDR-agonists and antagonists with high biological activity. Curr Topics Med Chem 2006; 6(12): 1273-1288; (c) Binderup L, Binderup E, Godtfredsen WO, Kissmeyer AM. Development of new vitamin D analogs. In Vitamin D (2nd Edition), Ed. Feldman D, Pike JW, Glorieux FH. 2005; 2: 1489-1510; (d) Peleg S, Posner GH. Vitamin D analogs as modulators of vitamin D receptor action. Curr Topics Med Chem 2003; 3(14): 1555-1572; (e) Zhu G-D, Okamura WH. Synthesis of Vitamin D (Calciferol). Chem Rev 1995; 95: 1877-1952.

[4] Tocchini-Valentini G, Rochel N, Wurtz JM, Mitschler A, Moras, D. Crystal structures of the vitamin D receptor complexed to superagonist 20-epi ligands. Proc Natl Acad Sci USA 2001; 98: 5491–5496.

[5] Vanhooke JL, Benning MM, Bauer CB, Pike JW, DeLuca HF. Molecular structure of the rat vitamin D receptor ligand binding domain complexed with 2-carbon-substituted vitamin D3 hormone analogues and a LXXLL-containing coactivator peptide. Biochemistry 2004; 43: 4101–4110.

[6] Uskokovic MR, Norman AW, Manchand PS, Studzinski GP, Campbell MJ, Koeffler HP, Takeuchi A, Siu-Caldera ML, Rao DS, Reddy GS. Steroids 2001; 66: 463-71.

[7] Rochel N, Moras D. Ligand biding domain of vitamin D receptors. Curr Topics Med Chem 2006; 6: 1229-1241.

[8] Rochel N, Moras D. Ligand biding domain of vitamin D receptors. Curr Topics Med Chem 2006; 6: 1229-1241.

[9] Brown AJ, Slatopolsky E. Drug Insight: vitamin D analogs in the treatment of secondary hyperparathyroidism in patients with chronic kidney disease. Endocr Metabol 2007; 3(2): 134-144.

[10] Kalantar-Zadeh K, Shah A, Duong U, Hechter RC, Dukkipati R, Kovesdy CP. Kidney bone disease and mortality in CKD: revisiting the role of vitamin D, calcimimetics, alkaline phosphatase, and minerals. Kidney Int 2010; 78 (suppl. 117): S10-S21.

[11] Kalantar-Zadeh K, Shah A, Duong U, Hechter RC, Dukkipati R, Kovesdy CP. Kidney bone disease and mortality in CKD: revisiting the role of vitamin D, calcimimetics, alkaline phosphatase, and minerals. Kidney Int 2010; 78 (suppl. 117): S10-S21.

[12] Luong QT, Koeffler HP. Vitamin D compounds in leukemia. Steroid Biochem Mol Biol 2005; 97: 195-202.

[13] Wu-Wong JR. Are vitamin D receptor activators useful for the treatment of thrombosis? Curr Opin Invest Drugs 2009; 10 (9): 919-927.

[14] http://www.iom.edu/Reports/2010/Dietary-Reference-Intakes-for-Calcium-and-Vitamin-D/DRI-Values.aspx.

[15] For a review, see: Norman AW, Bouillon R. Vitamin D nutritional policy needs a vision for the future. Exp Biol Med 2010, 235: 1034-1045.

[16] Houghton LA, Vieth R. The case against ergocalciferol (vitamin D2) as a vitamin supplement. Am J Clin Nutri 2006; 84(4): 694-7.

[17] Hackman KL, Gagnon C, Briscoe RK, Lam S, Anpalahan M, Ebeling P. Efficacy and safety of oral continuous low-dose versus short-term high-dose vitamin D: a prospective randomised trial conducted in a clinical setting. Med J Australia 2010; 192(12): 686-9.

[18] Nogues X, Servitja S, Pena MJ, Prieto-Alhambra D, Nadal R, Mellibovsky L, Albanell J, Diez-Perez A, Tusquets I. Vitamin D deficiency and bone mineral density in postmenopausal women receiving aromatase inhibitors for early breast cancer. Maturitas 2010; 66(3): 291-297.

[19] Garland CF, Garland FC. Do sunlight and vitamin D reduce the likelihood of colon cancer? Int J Epidemiol 1980; 9: 227–31.

[20] Amir E, Simmons C, Freedman C, Dranitsaris G, Cole DE, Vieth R, Ooi WS, Clemons M. A phase 2 trial exploring the effects of high-dose (10,000 IU/Day) vitamin D3 in breast cancer patients with bone metastases. Cancer 2010, 284-291.

[21] Garland CF, Gorham ED, Mohr SB, Grant WB, Giovannucci EL, Lipkin M, Newmark H, Holick MF, Garland FC. Vitamin D and prevention of breast cancer: pooled analysis. J Steroid Biochem Mol Biol 2007; 103: 708–11.

[22] http://www.urmc.rochester.edu/news/story/index.cfm?id=3013.

[23] http://www.mayoclinic.org/news2010-rst/6033.html?rss-feedid=1.

[24] IARC. Vitamin D and Cancer vol 5. IARC Working Group Reports, International Agency for Research on Cancer. Lyon: WHO, 2008.

[25] Giovannucci E, Liu Y, Hollis BW, Rimm EB. 25-Hydroxyvitamin D and Risk of Myocardial Infarction in Men: A Prospective Study. Arch Intern Med 2008; 168: 1174 – 1180.

[26] Melamed ML, Michos ED, Post W, Astor B. 25-hydroxyvitamin D levels and the risk of mortality in the general population. Arch Intern Med 2008; 168: 1629–37.

[27] Kovesdy CP, Ahmadzadeh S, Anderson JE, Kalantar-Zadeh K. Association of activated vitamin D treatment and mortality in chronic kidney disease. Arch Intern Med 2008; 168: 397–403.

[28] Wolf M, Betancourt J, Chang Y, Shah A, Teng M, Tamez H, Gutierrez O, Camargo CA Jr, Melamed M, Norris K, Stampfer MJ, Powe NR, Thadhani R. Impact of activated vitamin D and race on survival among hemodialysis patients. J Am Soc Nephrol 2008;19:1379–88.

[29] Bjorkman , Sorva A, Tilvis R. Responses of parathyroid hormone to vitamin D supplementation: A systematic review of clinical trials. Arch Gerontol Geriatrics 2009; 48(2): 160-166.

[30] Smolders J, Damoiseaux J, Menheere P, Hupperts R. Vitamin D as an immune modulator in multiple sclerosis, a review. J Neuroimmunol 2008; 194(1-2): 7-17.

[31] Hypponen E, Laara E, Reunanen A, Jarvelin MR, Virtanen SM. Intake of vitamin D and risk of type 1 diabetes: a birth-cohort study. Lancet 2001;358:1500–3.

[32] Mathieu C, Gysemans C, Giulietti A, Bouillon R. Vitamin D and diabetes. Diabetologia 2005; 49: 217–18.

[33] Burton JM, Kimball S, Vieth R, Bar-Or A, Dosch HM, Cheung R, Gagne D, D'Souza C, Ursell M, O'Connor P. A phase I/II dose-escalation trial of vitamin D3 and calcium in multiple sclerosis. Neurology 2010; 74(23): 1852-1859.

[34] Mowry EM, Krupp LB, Milazzo M, Chabas D, Strober JB, Belman AL, McDonald JC, Oksenberg JR, Bacchetti P, Waubant E. Vitamin D status is associated with relapse rate in pediatric-onset multiple sclerosis. Ann Neurol 2010; 67(5): 618-624.

[35] Skinner HG, Litzelman K, Schwartz GG. Recent clinical trials of vitamin D3 supplementation and serum calcium levels in humans: implications for vitamin D-based chemoprevention. Curr Opin Invest Drugs (BioMed Central) 2010; 11(6): 678-687.

[36] Orimo H, Schacht E. The D-hormone analog alfacalcidol: The pioneer beyond the horizon of osteoporosis treatment. J Rheumatol 2005; 32 (suppl. 76): 4-10.

[37] Hayashi Y, Fujita T, Inoue T. Decrease of vertebral fractures in osteoporosis by administration of 1-alpha-hydroxyvitamin D3. J Bone Miner Metab 1992; 10:50-4.

[38] Tanizawa T, Imura K, Ishii Y, *et al.* Treatment with active vitamin D metabolites and concurrent treatment in the prevention of hip fractures; a retrospective study. Osteoporosis Int 1999;9:163-70.

[39] Orimo H. Clinical application of 1 alpha (OH)D3 in Japan. Akt Rheumatol 1994;19:27.

[40] Ringe JD, Dorst A, Faber H, Schacht E, Rahlfs VW. Superiority of alfacalcidol over plain vitamin D in the treatment of glucocorticoid-induced osteoporosis. Rheumatol Int 2004;24:63-70.

[41] Ringe JD, Schacht E. Potential of alfacalcidol for reducing increased risk of falls and fractures. Rheumatol Int 2009; 29(10): 1177-1185.

[42]   Jean-Yves R, Marie-Paule L, Florent R. Importance of alfacalcidol in clinical conditions characterized by high rate of bone loss. J Rheumatol Supplement 2005; 76: 21-5.

[43]   Patel TV, Singh AK. Does treatment with calcitriol improve survival in predialysis patients with chronic kidney disease? Nature Clinical Practice 2008; 4(9): 484-485.

[44]   Rizova E, Corroller M. Topical calcitriol--studies on local tolerance and systemic safety. Br J Dermatol 2001; 144 (Suppl 58): 3-10.

[45]   Beer TM, Garzotto M, Park B, Mori M, Myrthue A, Janeba N, Sauer D, Eilers K. Effect of calcitriol on prostate-specific antigen *in vitro* and in humans. Clin Cancer Res 2006; 12(9): 2812-2816.

[46]   Finlay IG, Stewart GJ, Ahkter J, Morris DL. A phase one study of the hepatic arterial administration of 1,25-dihydroxyvitamin D3 for liver cancers. J Gastroenterol Hepatol 2001; 16(3): 333-337.

[47]   Yu WD, Ma Y, Flynn G, Muindi JR, Kong RX, Trump DL, Johnson CS. Calcitriol enhances gemcitabine anti-tumor activity *in vitro* and *in vivo* by promoting apoptosis in a human pancreatic carcinoma model system. Cell Cycle 2010; 9(15): 3022-9.

[48]   Griffin MD, Kumar R. Multiple potential clinical benefits for 1alpha,25-dihydroxyvitamin D3 analogs in kidney transplant recipients. J Steroid Biochem Mol Biol 2005; 97(1-2): 213-8.

[49]   Dennis V, Albertson GL. Doxercalciferol treatment of secondary hyperparathyroidism. Ann Pharmacother 2006; 40: 1955-1965.

[50]   Zisman AL, Ghantous W, Schinleber P, Roberts L. Inhibition of parathyroid hormone: a dose equivalency study of paricalcitol and doxercalciferol. Am J Nephrol 2005; 25: 591-595.

[51]   Moe SM, Saifullah A, LaClair RE, Usman SA, Yu Z. A randomized trial of cholecalciferol versus doxercalciferol for lowering parathyroid hormone in chronic kidney disease. Clin J Am Soc Nephrol 2010; 5(2): 299-306.

[52]   Liu G, Wilding G, Staab MJ, Horvath D, Miller K, Dresen A, Alberti D, Arzoomanian R, Chappell R, Bailey HH. Phase II Study of 1α-Hydroxyvitamin D_2 in the Treatment of Advanced Androgen-independent Prostate Cancer Clin Cancer Res 2003; 9(11): 4077-4083.

[53]   Wanyoike GN, Shigeyama T, Nagai H, Toyoda A. Method for producing crystals of vitamin D derivative. WO2010/095425A1.

[54]   Souza FES, Pan M, Turcot KDS. Paricalcitol purification. US 2010/0063307.

[55]   Schroeder NJ, Burrin JM, Noonan K. Effects of 'non- calcaemic' vitamin D analogues on 24-hydroxylase expression in MG-63 osteoblast-like cells. Nephron Physiol 2003; 94 (4): 62-73.

[56]   Slatopolsky E, Cozzolino M, Lu Y. Efficacy of 19-Nor- 1,25-(OH)2D2 in the prevention and treatment of hyperparathyroid bone disease in experimental uremia. Kidney Int 2003; 63 (6): 2020-2027.

[57]   Takahashi F, Finch JL, Denda M, *et al.* A new analog of 1,25- (OH)2D3, 19-NOR-1,25-(OH)2D2, suppresses serum PTH and parathyroid gland growth in uremic rats without elevation of intestinal vitamin D receptor content. Am J Kidney Dis 1997; 30 (1): 105-112.

[58]   Nakane M, Fey TA, Dixon DB. Effect of vitamin D receptor activators on bone formation and resorption [abstract no. SA PO611]. Proceedings of the American Society of Nephrology; 2004 Oct 27-Nov 1; St Louis.

[59]   Robinson DM, Scott LJ. Paricalcitol, a review of its use in the management of secondary hyperparathyroidism. Drugs 2005; 65(4): 559-576.

[60]   Martin KJ, Gonzalez EA, Gellens M, *et al.* 19-Nor-1-□-25-dihydroxyvitamin D2 (Paricalcitol) safely and effectively reduces the levels of intact parathyroid hormone in patients on hemodialysis. J Am Soc Nephrol 1998; 9 (8): 1427-1432.

[61]   Llach F, Keshav G, Goldblat MV, *et al.* Suppression of parathy-roid hormone secretion in hemodialysis patients by a novel vitamin D analogue: 19-nor-1,25-dihydroxyvitamin D2. Am J Kidney Dis 1998; 32 (4 Suppl. 2): S48-54.

[62]   Abdul Gafor AH, Saidin R, Loo CY, Mohd R, Zainudin S, Shah SA, Norella KC Intravenous calcitriol versus paricalcitol in haemodialysis patients with severe secondary hyperparathyroidism. Nephrology (Carlton). 2008-2009; 14(5):488-92.

[63]   Nuijten M, Andress DL, Marx SE, Sterz R. Chronic kidney disease Markov model comparing paricalcitol to calcitriol for secondary hyperparathyroidism: a US perspective. Curr Med Res Opin 2009; 25(5): 1221-1234.

[64]   Lund RJ, Andress DL, Amdahl M, Williams LA, Heaney RP Differential effects of paricalcitol and calcitriol on intestinal calcium absorption in hemodialysis patients. Am J Nephrol 2010; 31(2):165-70.

[65]   Fishbane S, Chittineni H, Packman M, Dutka P, Ali N, Durie N. Oral paricalcitol in the treatment of patients with CKD and proteinuria: a randomized trial. Am J Kidney Dis 2009-2010; 54(4):647-52.

[66] de Zeeuw D, Agarwal R, Amdahl M, Audhya P, Coyne D, Garimella T, Parving HH, Pritchett Y, Remuzzi G, Ritz E, Andress D. Selective vitamin D receptor activation with paricalcitol for reduction of albuminuria in patients with type 2 diabetes (VITAL study): a randomised controlled trial. Lancet 2010; 376: 1543-1551.

[67] Koeffler HP, Aslanian N, O'Kelly J. Vitamin D2 analog (Paricalcitol; Zemplar) for treatment of myelodysplastic syndrome. Leukemia Research 2005; 29(11): 1259-1262.

[68] Kumagai T, Koeffler HP. Paricalcitol: a vitamin D2 analog with anticancer effects with low calcemic activity. New Topics Vitamin D Res 2006; 169-179.

[69] Alborzi P, Patel NA, Peterson C, Bills JE, Bekele DM, Bunaye Z, Light RP, Agarwal R. Paricalcitol reduces albuminuria and inflammation in chronic kidney disease: a randomized double-blind pilot trial. Hypertension 2008; 52(2):249-55.

[70] Tan X, He W, Liu Y.Combination therapy with paricalcitol and trandolapril reduces renal fibrosis in obstructive nephropathy. Kidney Int (2009), 76, 1248-1257.

[71] Kim TH, Ji JD. Paricalcitol, a synthetic vitamin D analog: A candidate for combination therapy with biological agents in rheumatoid arthritis. Medical Hypotheses 2010; 75(6): 634-635.

[72] Husain K, Suarez E, Isidro A, Ferder L. Effects of Paricalcitol and Enalapril on Atherosclerotic Injury in Mouse Aortas. Am J Nephr 2010; 32(4): 296-304.

[73] Van de Kerkhof P, de Peuter R, Ryttov J, *et al.* Mixed treatment comparison of a two-compound formulation (TCF) product containing calcipotriol and betamethasone dipropionate with other topical treatments in psoriasis vulgaris. Curr Med Res Opin 2011; 27:225-38.

[74] Freeman K. The two-compound formulation of calcipotriol and betamethasone dipropionate for treatment of moderately severe body and scalp psoriasis – an introduction. Curr Med Res Opin 2011; 27:197-203.

[75] Bottomley JM, Taylor RS, Ryttov J. The effectiveness of two-compound formulation calcipotriol and betamethasone dipropionate gel in the treatment of moderately severe scalp psoriasis: A systematic review of direct and indirect evidence. Curr Med Res Opin 2011; 27: 251-268.

[76] Guenther LC. Calcipotriene plus betamethasone dipropionate gel: a new combination therapy for scalp psoriasis. Expert Rev Dermatol 2009; 4(2): 111-118.

[77] Guenther L, Cambazard F, Van De Kerkhof PCM, Snellman E, Kragballe K, Chu AC, Tegner E, Garcia-Diez A, Springborg J. Efficacy and safety of a new combination of calcipotriol and betamethasone dipropionate (once or twice daily) compared to calcipotriol (twice daily) in the treatment of psoriasis vulgaris: a randomized, double-blind, vehicle-controlled clinical trial. Br J Dermat 2002; 147(2): 316-323.

[78] Langley RGB, Gupta A, Papp K, Wexler D, Østerdal ML, Ćurčić D. Calcipotriol plus Betamethasone Dipropionate Gel Compared with Tacalcitol Ointment and the Gel Vehicle Alone in Patients with Psoriasis Vulgaris: A Randomized, Controlled Clinical Trial. Dermatology 2011; 222(2): 148-156.

[79] Holm EA, Jemec GBE. The therapeutic potential of calcipotriol in diseases other than psoriasis. Int J Dermat 2002; 41(1): 38-43.

[80] van der Veer WM, Jacobs XE, Waardenburg IE, Ulrich MM, Niessen FB. Topical Calcipotriol for Preventive Treatment of Hypertrophic Scars. Arch Dermatol 2009; 145(11):1269-1275.

[81] Colston KW, Pirianov G, Bramm E, Hamberg KJ, Binderup L. Effects of Seocalcitol (EB1089) on nitrosomethyl urea-induced rat mammary tumors. Breast Cancer Res Treat 2003;80(3):303-11.

[82] Hansen CM, Hamberg KJ, Binderup E, Binderup L. Seocalcitol (EB 1089): a vitamin D analogue of anti-cancer potential. Background, design, synthesis, pre-clinical and clinical evaluation. Curr Pharmac Design 2000; 6(7): 803-828.

[83] Nuclear Receptors as Therapeutic Targets - Society for Medicines Research Symposium London, UK. *IDdb Meeting Report* (1999) September 16.

[84] Chaudhry M, Sundaram S, Gennings C, Carter H, Gewirtz DA. The vitamin D3 analog, ILX-23-7553, enhances the response to adriamycin and irradiation in MCF-7 breast tumor cells. Cancer Chemother Pharmacol 2001; 47(5): 429-36.

[85] Sundaram S, Sea A, Feldman S, Strawbridge R, Hoopes PJ, Demidenko E, Binderup L, Gewirtz, DA. The combination of a potent vitamin D analog, EB-1089, with ionizing radiation reduces tumor growth and induces apoptosis of MCF-7 breast tumor xenografts in nude mice. Clin Cancer Res 2003; 9: 2350-2356.

[86] Gewirtz DA, Gupta MS, DeMasters G, Park M, Gennings C, Jones K, Feldman S, Sea A, Strawbridge R, Hoopes J, Sundaram S: Selective (p53 dependent) promotion of apoptosis by the combination of the vitamin D3 analog EB1089 and fractionated radiation in MCF-7 breast tumor cells and in breast tumor cell xenografts. Proc Am Assoc Cancer Res 2003; 44: Abs R680.

[87]   Evans TJR, Colston KW, Lofts FJ, Cunningham D, Anthoney DA, Gogas H, de Bono JS, Hamberg KJ, Skov T, Mansi JL. A phase II trial of the vitamin D analogue Seocalcitol (EB1089) in patients with inoperable pancreatic cancer. Br J Cancer 2002; 86: 680–685.

[88]   Zhang X, Jiang F, Li P, Li C, Ma Q, Nicosia SV, Bai W. Growth suppression of ovarian cancer xenografts in nude mice by vitamin D analogue EB1089. Clin Cancer Res 2005; 11: 323-328.

[89]   Dalhoff K, Dancey J, Astrup L, Skovsgaard T, Hamberg KJ, Lofts FJ, Rosmorduc O, Erlinger S, Bach Hansen J, Steward WP, Skov T, Burcharth F, Evans TR. A phase II study of the vitamin D analogue seocalcitol in patients with inoperable hepatocellular carcinoma. Br J Cancer 2003; 89(2): 252-257.

[90]   Evans TR, Colston KW, Lofts FJ, Cunningham D, Anthoney DA, Gogas H, de Bono JS, Hamberg KJ, Skov T, Mansi JL. A phase II trial of the vitamin D analogue seocalcitol (EB1089) in patients with inoperable pancreatic cancer. Br J Cancer 2002; 86(5):680-685.

[91]   Harrison PV. Topical tacalcitol treatment for psoriasis. Hosp Med 2000; 61: 402-5.

[92]   Gollnick H, Menke T. Current experience with tacalcitol ointment in the treatment of psoriasis. Curr Med Res Opin 1998; 14: 213-8.

[93]   Leone G, Pacifico A. Profile of clinical efficacy and safety of topical tacalcitol. Acta Bio-medica: Atenei Parmensis 2005; 76: 13-19.

[94]   Kokelj F, Plozzer C, Guadagnini A.Topical tacalcitol reduces the total UVB dosage in the treatment of psoriasis vulgaris. J Dermatol Treat 1996; 7: 265-6.

[95]   Katayama I, Ashida M, Maeda A, Eishi K, Murota H, Bae SJ. Open trial of topical tacalcitol and solar irradiation for vitiligo vulgaris:upregulation of c-Kit mRNA by cultured melanocytes. Eur J Dermatol 2003; 13: 372-6.

[96]   Leone G, Pacifico A, Iacovelli P, Paro Vidolin A, Picardo M. Tacalcitol and narrow-band phototherapy in patients with vitiligo. Clin Exp Dermatol 2006; 31(2): 200-5.

[97]   Tang L, Fu W, Xiang L, Jin Y, ZhengZ. Topical tacalcitol and 308-nm monochromatic excimer light: a synergistic combination for the treatment of vitiligo. Photodermatology, Photoimmunology & Photomedicine 2006; 22: 310-314.

[98]   Rodriguez-Martin M, Bustinduy MG, Rodriguez MS, Cabrera AN. Randomized, double-blind clinical trial to evaluate the efficacy of topical tacalcitol and sunlight exposure in the treatment of adult nonsegmental vitiligo. Br J Dermatol 2009: 160(2): 409-414.

[99]   Hayashi J, Matsui C, Mitsuishi T, Kawashima M, Morohashi M. Treatment of localized epidermodysplasia verruciformis with tacalcitol ointment. Int J Dermatol 2002; 41: 817-20.

[100]   Hayashi H. Treatment of Grover's disease with tacalcitol. Clin Exp Dermatol 2002; 27: 160-5.

[101]   Shimizu H, Shimizu K, Kubodera N, Mikami T, Tsuzaki K, Suwa H, Harada K, Hiraide A, Shimizu M, KoyamaK, Ichikawa Y, Hirasawa Y, Kito D, Kobayashi M, Kigawa M, Kato M, Kozono T, Tanaka H, Tanabe M, Iguchi M, Yoshida M. Industrial Synthesis of Maxacalcitol, the Antihyperparathyroidism and Antipsoriatic Vitamin D3 Analogue Exhibiting Low Calcemic Activity. Org Process Res Devel 2005; 9: 278-287.

[102]   Brown A, Slatopolsky E. Drug insight: vitamin D analogs in the treatment of secondary hyperparathyroidism in patients with chronic kidney disease. Nature Clin Practice 2007; 3(2) 134-144.

[103]   Hayashi1 M, Tsuchiya Y, Itaya Y, Takenaka T, Kobayashi K. Yoshizawa M, Nakamura R, Monkawa T, Ichihara1 A. Comparison of the effects of calcitriol and maxacalcitol on secondary hyperparathyroidism in patients on chronic haemodialysis: a randomized prospective multicentre trial. Nephrol Dial Transplant 2004; 19: 2067–2073.

[104]   Shiizaki K, Hatamura I, Nakazawa E, Ogura M, Masuda T, Akizawa T, Kusano E. Review: Molecular and morphological approach of uremia-induced hyperplastic parathyroid gland following direct maxacalcitol injection. Med Mol Morphol 2008; 41(2): 76-82.

[105]   Barker JN, Ashton RE, Marks R, Harris RI, Berth-Jones J. Topical maxacalcitol for the treatment of psoriasis vulgaris: a placebo-controlled, double-blind, dose-finding study with active comparator. Br J Dermatol 1999; 141(2): 274-278.

[106]   Umemura K, Ikeda Y, Kondo K, Hirata K, Amagishi H, Ishihama Y, Tokura Y. Cutaneous pharmacokinetics of topically applied maxacalcitol ointment and lotion. Int J Clin Pharmacol Ther 2008; 46(6): 289-94.

[107]   Abe M, Syuto T, Hasegawa M, Yokoyama Y, Ishikawa O. Clinical usefulness of a supplementary cyclosporin administration with a topical application of maxacalcitol ointment for patients with moderate psoriasis vulgaris. J Dermatol 2009; 36(4): 197-201.

[108]   Imagawa I, Suzuki H. Successful treatment of refractory warts with topical vitamin D_3 derivative (maxacalcitol, 1a,25-dihydroxy-2-oxacalcitriol) in 17 patients. J Dermatol 2007; 34: 264-266.

[109]   Kimura M, Higuchi T, Yoshida M. Infantile Acropustulosis Treated Successfully With Topical Maxacalcitol. Acta Derm Venereol 2011; 91: 1-2.

[110] de Jager MEA, de Jong EMGJ, van de Kerkhof PCM, Seyger, MMB. Efficacy and safety of treatments for childhood psoriasis: a systematic literature review. J Am Acad Dermatol 2010; 62(6): 1013-1030.

[111] Morii H. Falecalcitriol as a new therapeutic agent for secondary hyperparathyroidism. Clin Calcium 2005;15(1): 29-33.

[112] Nishizawa Y, et al. 26,26,26,27,27,27-hexafluoro-1,25-dihydroxyvitamin D3 in uremic patients on hemodialysis: preliminary report. Contrib Nephrol 1991; 90: 196-203.

[113] Ito H, Ogata H, Yamamoto M, Takahashi K, Shishido K, Takahashi J, Taguchi S, Kinugasa E. Comparison of oral falecalcitriol and intravenous calcitriol in hemodialysis patients with secondary hyperparathyroidism: a randomized, crossover trial. Clin Nephrol 2009; 71(6): 660-8.

[114] Noboru O, Koji U. Pharmacological action and clinical effects of falecalcitriol, a highly potent derivative of active vitamin D$_3$. Folia Pharmacologica Japonica 2002; 120(6): 427-36.

[115] Tokunaga M, Tamura M, Kabashima N, Serino R, Shibata T, Matsumoto M, Miyamoto T, Miyazaki M, Furuno Y, Takeuchi M, Abe H, Okazaki M, Otsuji Y. Falecalcitriol for conventional vitamin D therapy-resistant secondary hyperparathyroidism in a continuous ambulatory peritoneal dialysis patient. Clin Nephr 2008; 69(5): 393-4.

[116] Brown W. Vitamin D, vitamin D analogs (deltanoids) and prostate cancer. Expert Rev Clin Pharmacol 2008; 1(6): 803-813.

[117] Ahmed I. ED-71 (Chugai). Curr Opinion Invest Drugs 2004; 5(4): 441-447.

[118] Tsuji N, Takahashi F. Therapeutic agents for disorders of bone and calcium metabolism. ED-71 Clinical Calcium 2007; 17(1): 72-79.

[119] Matsumoto T. New active vitamin D, ED-71, increases bone mass in osteoporotic patients under vitamin D supplementation: a randomized, double-blind, placebo-controlled clinical trial. J Clin Endocrinol Metab 2005; 90: 5031–5036.

[120] Matsumoto T, Kubodera N. ED-71, a new active vitamin D3, increases bone mineral density regardless of serum 25(OH)D levels in osteoporotic subjects. J. Steroid Biochem Mol Biol 2007; 103(3-5): 584-586.

[121] Peleg S, Uskokovic M, Ahene A, Vickery B, Avnur Z. Cellular and molecular events associated with the bone-protecting activity of the noncalcemic vitamin D analog Ro-26-9228 in osteopenic rats. Endocrinology 2002; 143(5): 1625-36.

[122] Revill P, Serradell N. Elocalcitol. Drugs of the Future 2006; 31(12): 1042-1047.

[123] Tiwari A. Elocalcitol (BXL-628): a novel, investigational therapy for the therapeutic management of benign prostatic hyperplasia. Expert Opin Inbestig Drugs 2008; 17(5): 819-823.

[124] Atul T. Elocalcitol, a vitamin D3 analog for the potential treatment of benign prostatic hyperplasia, overactive bladder and male infertility. IDrugs: the investigational drugs journal 2009; 12(6): 381-93.

[125] BioXell news release: http://www.tvm-capital.com/pages/news/2009/bio0428.php.

[126] Posner GH, Wang Q, Han G, Lee JK, Crawford K, Zand S, Brem H, Peleg S, Dolan P, Kensler TW. Conceptually new sulfone analogues of the hormone 1alpha, 25-dihydroxyvitamin D3: synthesis and preliminary biological evaluation. J Med Chem 1999; 42 (18): 3425–3435.

[127] Posner G, Helvig C, Cuerrier D, Collop D, Kharebov A, Ryder K, Epps T, Petkovich M. Vitamin D analogues targeting CYP24 in chronic kidney disease J Steroid Biochem Mol Biol 2010; 121: 13-19.

[128] http://www.drugs.com/clinical_trials/cytochroma-announces-positive-comparative-data-cta018-6105.html.

[129] Sicinski RR, Prahl JM, Smith CM, DeLuca HF. New 1alpha,25-dihydroxy-19-norvitamin D3 compounds of high biological activity: synthesis and biological evaluation of 2-hydroxymethyl, 2-methyl, and 2-methylene analogues. J Med Chem. 1998; 41: 4662–4674.

[130] Shevde NK, Plum LA, Clagett-Dame M, Yamamoto H, Pike JW, DeLuca HF. A potent analog of 1alpha, 25-dihydroxyvitamin D3 selectively induces bone formation. Proc Natl Acad Sci USA 2002; 99: 13487–13491.

[131] Ke HZ, Qi H, Crawford DT, et al. A new vitamin D analog, 2MD, restores trabecular and cortical bone mass and strength in ovariectomized rats with established osteopenia. J Bone Miner Res 2005; 20: 1742–1755.

[132] Plum LA, Fitzpatrick LA, Ma X, et al. 2MD, a new anabolic agent for osteoporosis treatment. Osteoporos Int 2006;17:704–715.

[133] DeLuca HF, Bedale W, Binkley N, Gallagher JC, Bolognese M, Peacock M, Aloia J, Clagett-Dame M, Plum L. The vitamin D analogue 2MD increases bone turnover but not BMD in postmenopausal women with osteopenia: results of a 1-year phase 2 double-blind, placebo-controlled, randomized clinical trial. J Bone Min Res 2011; 26(3): 538-545.

Vitamin D and Your Body, 2012, 83-101

CHAPTER 6

How are Vitamin D and Its Analogs Used to Treat Human Diseases?

Alex J. Brown*

Renal Division, Washington University School of Medicine, USA

Abstract: The vitamin D endocrine system was originally discovered for its critical role in calcium and phosphate homeostasis. The active form of vitamin D, 1,25-dihydroxyvitamin D_3 (calcitriol), promotes intestinal absorption of calcium and phosphate, but actions on bone, kidney and the parathyroids also contribute to the control of mineral metabolism. Subsequently, the vitamin D receptor (VDR) was detected in many other target tissues where calcitriol exerts pleiotropic effects, often in an autocrine/paracrine fashion. These non-classical activities of calcitriol have suggested therapeutic applications of calcitriol for the treatment of hyperproliferative disorders (*e.g.* cancer and psoriasis), immune dysfunction (autoimmune diseases), and endocrine disorders (*e.g.* hyperparathyroidism). In many cases, however, the effective therapeutic doses of calcitriol are hypercalcemic, a limitation that has spurred the development of vitamin D analogs that retain the therapeutically useful actions of calcitriol, but with reduced calcemic activity. Analogs with wider therapeutic windows are available for treatment of psoriasis and secondary hyperparathyroidism in chronic kidney disease, and research on even more effective analogs for these indications continues. Pre-clinical and clinical trials of analogs for treatment of several types of cancer, autoimmune disorders, and many other diseases are underway. Newer analogs show promise in various cellular models, but this review will focus on analogs currently in use and those with documented efficacy in animal models or in clinical trials.

Keywords: Autoimmune diseases, breast cancer, colon cancer, leukemia, osteoporosis, pancreatic cancer, prostate cancer, psoriasis, secondary hyperparathyroidism, skin cancer, transplant rejection.

INTRODUCTION

Vitamin D was discovered as a key regulator of calcium and phosphate homeostasis through actions on the intestine, kidney, bone and parathyroid glands. Vitamin D_3 (cholecalciferol) is made in the skin by ultraviolet photolysis of 7-dehyrocholesterol and must be activated by two successive hydroxylations at Carbon 25 and 1 to the activated, hormonal form: 1,25-dihydroxyvitamin D_3 (calcitriol). Vitamin D_2 (ergocalciferol), obtained from the diet (fish oil, mushrooms) and from supplements, is also activated to 1,25-dihydroxyvitamin D_2, which is similar in activity to calcitriol. Most of the actions of calcitriol are mediated by the vitamin D receptor (VDR) [1]. Calcitriol regulates mineral homeostasis by activation of the VDR in the intestine, kidney, bone and parathyroid glands. However, the VDR is present in many other tissues, where it mediates cell-specific actions of calcitriol that are unrelated to mineral metabolism. Many of these "non-classical" actions, including inhibition of cell proliferation, modulation of the immune system, and control or other hormones and cytokines, have suggested potential roles for calcitriol in control of disorders such as cancer, autoimmune diseases. However, these potential therapeutic applications of calcitriol are often precluded by the potent calcemic and phosphatemic effects of the native vitamin D hormone. This led to development of vitamin D analogs with more selective actions, *i.e.*, greater therapeutic activity with less hypercalcemia and hyperphosphatemia. This chapter reviews the analogs that have been found to be effective therapeutics in clinical and preclinical studies. Several are now approved for use in patients. The analogs will be designated by their chemical and generic names. For reference, please see previous chapters for the numbering of the carbon atoms in the vitamin D backbone. In this chapter potential therapeutic indications for vitamin D analogs will be discussed by indication. For this purpose, although previous chapters (especially Chapter 5) have illustrated the structures of several vitamin D analogs currently on the market or in development, the structures of additional vitamin D analogs discussed in this chapter are provided in Fig. **1**.

---

*Address correspondence to Alex J. Brown:** Department of Medicine, Washington University School of Medicine, St. Louis, MO, 63130, USA; E-mail: ABROWN@DOM.wustl.edu

J. Ruth Wu-Wong (Ed)

THERAPEUTIC APPLICATIONS OF VITAMIN D ANALOGS

Currently vitamin D analogs are available for treatment of osteoporosis, psoriasis and secondary hyperparathyroidism in chronic kidney disease, and data exist to suggest the expansion of usage to other diseases.

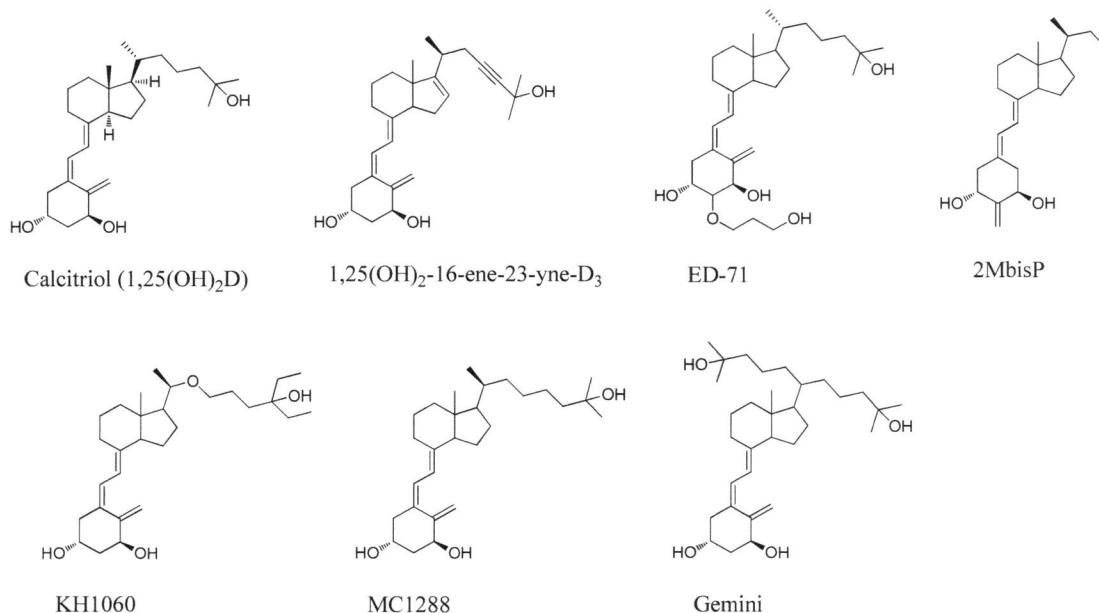

Calcitriol (1,25(OH)$_2$D)   1,25(OH)$_2$-16-ene-23-yne-D$_3$ ED-71   2MbisP

KH1060   MC1288   Gemini

Figure 1: Structures of calcitriol and selected analogs.

PSORIASIS

The pathogenesis of psoriasis is not completely understood, but appears to be mediated by Th1 cells and involves keratinocyte hyperproliferation. The immunosuppressive and anti-inflammatory properties of active vitamin D compounds led to the successful application of calcitriol, but less calcemic analogs provide a greater safety margin, especially when large areas are treated.

Calcipotriol, the first analog to be introduced for psoriasis (see the structure in the previous chapter), has the same VDR affinity as calcitriol, and retains its abilities to terminally differentiate proliferating keratinocytes [2] and to modulate keratinocyte release of immune mediators *in vitro* [3, 4]. On the other hand, calcipotriol was more than 200 times less calcemic and calciuric in rats [5]. In patients, topical calcipotriol was effective in reducing psoriatic lesions. Hypercalcemia was minimal since the analog is poorly aborbed into the blood [6]. Calcipotriol is now widely used for treatment of psoriasis in Europe and the United States.

Other vitamin D analogs have been shown to be effective for psoriasis. Topical tacalcitol (1,24(OH)$_2$D$_3$) [7] inhibits keratinocyte proliferation as effectively as calcitriol [8], but with nearly the same calcemic activity, indicating its therapeutic window may be similar. 22-Oxa-calcitriol (maxacalcitol) is more active than calcitriol in terminally differentiating keratinocytes *in vitro* [9], but less calcemic *in vivo*. Maxacalcitol was effective in clinical trials [10] and is currently available in Japan for treatment of psoriasis.

SECONDARY HYPERPARATHYROIDISM (SHPT, 2°HPT) IN CHRONIC KIDNEY DISEASE

Secondary hyperparathyroidism (SHPT) is common in patients with chronic kidney disease (CKD). The pathogensis of SHPT is diagrammed in Fig. **2**. The primary factor responsible for high PTH is a decrease in serum calcium, due to hyperphosphatemia which complexes serum free calcium levels and to reduced renal production of calcitriol which leads to decreased intestinal calcium absorption [11]. Reduced calcitriol also can increase PTH directly, as the vitamin D hormone is a repressor of PTH gene transcription. Hyperphosphatemia also has a direct stimulatory effect on PTH synthesis. In addition, hyperphosphatemia can stimulate increase serum fibroblast growth factor 23 (FGF-23), a potent inhibitor of calcitriol production, as well as PTH [12]. With chronic stimulation, the parathyroid glands eventually become hyperplastic to increase PTH secretory capacity.

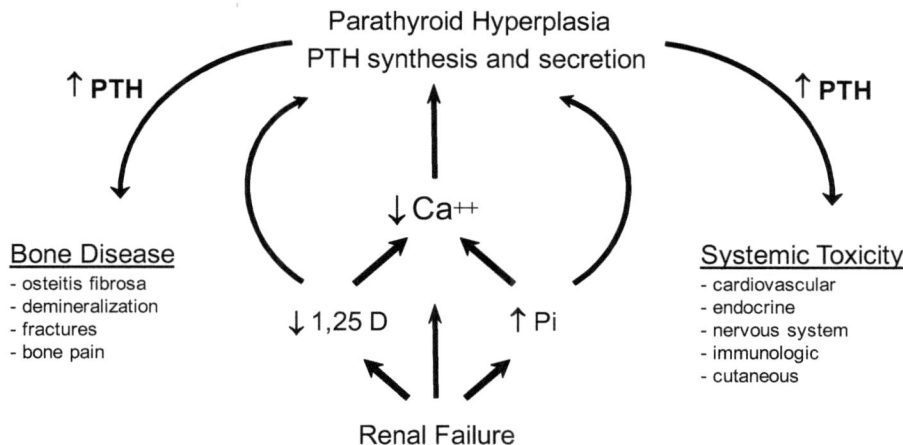

Figure 2: The pathogenesis of secondary hyperparathyroidism in chronic kidney disease and the role of vitamin D therapy. Loss of renal function leads to phosphate (Pi) retention and a decrease in serum calcitriol ($1,25(OH)_2D$), both of which reduce serum calcium levels. Hypocalcemia stimulates the PTH synthesis and secretion and, eventually, parathyroid gland hyperplasia. The effects of hyperparathyroidism on bone and other tissues are listed.

The chronically high PTH levels in patients with CKD produce a state of high turnover bone and osteitis fibrosa. The poorly formed (woven) bone and loss of bone mineral lead to microfractures and pain [13, 14]. In addition, calcium and phosphate released from the skeleton contribute to vascular calcification and coronary artery disease, the leading cause of death in CKD patients [13]. While treatment with calcitriol or its pro-drug precursor $1\alpha(OH)D_3$ (alfacalcidol) has been shown to be generally effective in reducing PTH levels, the potent calcemic effects of calcitriol, primarily from stimulation of intestinal calcium absorption, results in a relatively narrow therapeutic window. In addition, calcium supplements are often used to reduce phosphate absorption by CKD patients. This increases the risk of hypercalcemia and over-suppression of PTH, leading to low turnover or adynamic bone disease, which impairs the buffering capacity of the bone, ultimately increasing vascular calcification [13]. These limitations of calcitriol for treatment of SHPT prompted the search for vitamin D analogs with wider therapeutic windows. At present, four vitamin D analogs have been approved for treatment of SHPT in CKD patients, and several others are in development.

Maxacalcitol (22-Oxa-calcitriol) was the first analog found to have a wider therapeutic window than calcitriol in suppressing PTH. This analog retained very high potency to suppress PTH *in vitro* and *in vivo* [15], but was much less calcemic than calcitriol [16]. In animal models of CKD, maxacalcitol was slightly less active than calcitriol in reducing PTH, but had much lower calcemic activity [17-20]. Analysis of bone from uremic rats, showed that maxacalcitol could restore normal bone metabolism [20, 21].

The efficacy of maxacalcitol was demonstrated in hemodialysis patients [22-26], although hypercalcemia was observed with higher doses [24]. Intravenous maxacalcitol was comparable to oral calcitriol over 24 weeks in both suppressing PTH levels and in hypercalcemic episodes [22]. Other trials examining intravenous maxacalcitol versus intravenous calcitriol found comparable efficacies and safety [26], but maxacalcitol was more effective in reducing markers of bone turnover [27]. Maxacalcitol is currently available in Japan for patients who have CKD with SHPT.

Paricalcitol (19-nor-$1,25(OH)_2D_2$) was the first of less calcemic vitamin D analogs to be approved for SHPT. This analog lacks carbon 19 in the A-ring and has the vitamin D_2 side chain instead of the vitamin

D_3 side chain of calcitriol (see Table **2** in Chapter 5). Paricalcitol was shown to be 10 times less calcemic and phosphatemic than calcitriol, but only about 3 times less active in suppressing PTH [28]. Non-calcemic doses of paricalcitol prevented parathyroid gland hyperplasia [29] and high turnover bone disease in uremic rats [30]. In addition, less vascular calcification was observed with paricalcitol than with calcitriol [31] or $1\alpha(OH)D_2$ [32, 33]. The mechanisms responsible for these differences are not known.

Intravenous paricalcitol effectively reduced PTH in hemodialysis patients with few episodes of hypercalcemia [34, 35]. As in uremic rats, paricalcitol was about three times less potent than calcitriol in suppressing PTH [35], but few direct comparisons of paricalcitol with calcitriol or other analogs have been carried out. However, in one dose-escalation study, paricalcitol reduced PTH more rapidly than calcitriol with fewer hypercalcemic episodes [36]. Paricalcitol is now available in the U.S.A. and Europe in both intravenous and oral forms.

Doxercalciferol $(1\alpha(OH)D_2)$ is a synthetic precursor of 1,25-dihydroxyvitamin D_2, and must be activated by 25-hydroxylation, primarily in the liver (see Chapter 5). It is less calcemic than its D_3 counterpart alfacalicol $(1\alpha(OH)D_3)$ [37]. After an unsuccessful trial for treatment of osteoporosis, the efficacy of doxercalciferol to control SHPT was assessed in dialysis patients. Several studies found that oral doxercalciferol could effectively reduce PTH levels, but mild hypercalcemia was observed overall and the frequency of hypercalcemic episodes was greater than during washout [38, 39]. Similar efficacy of oral doxercalciferol was demonstrated in pre-dialysis patients [40]. More recently, an intravenous formulation of doxercalciferol was approved for dialysis patients.

Direct comparisons of the selectivity of analogs for SHPT are very limited. In uremic rats, doxercalciferol was found to be generally more active than paricalcitol, but relative therapeutic windows were not determined [41]. In separate studies in patients, doxercalciferol was found to be nearly twice as active as paricalcitol in suppressing PTH [42], and about 10 times more potent in mobilizing calcium from bone [43]. Further studies would be required to determine the relative selectivities of these two compounds [44].

Falecalcitriol $(1,25(OH)_2\text{-}26,27\text{-}F_6\text{-}D_3)$ (see Chapter 5) is the most recent analog to be for SHPT in Japan. The fluoro substitutions impede catabolism of falecalcitriol, rendering it more active than calcitriol *in vivo* [45]. In fact, the 23-hydroxy metabolite of falecalcitriol, which retains considerable activity, accumulates in target tissues, including both the parathyroid glands and the intestine [46]. Thus, it is unlikely that the analog is selective in suppressing PTH. Clinical studies were not impressive with a very modest reduction in PTH at non-calcemic doses and marginal superiority to alfacalcidol [47]. A direct comparison to calcitriol revealed no advantage of falecalcitriol [48].

A number of other analogs have been assessed in the uremic rat model for efficacy in treating SHPT. These include $1,25(OH)_2$-dihydrotachysterol [49], three 20-epi analogs from Leo Pharmaceuticals (CB1093, EB1213 and GS1725) [50], $1,25(OH)_2$-16-ene,23-yne-D_3 (Fig. **1**) [51], $1\alpha(OH)$-3-epi-D_3 [52] and (20S)-1α-hydroxy-2-methylene-19-nor-bishomopregnacalciferol (2MbisP) [53, 54]. However, no clinical studies have been reported for these analogs in the treatment of SHPT.

SURVIVAL IN CHRONIC KIDNEY DISEASE

Analysis of large databases of dialysis patients revealed that treatment with calcitriol or its analogs can reduce morbidity and mortality in CKD patients through mechanisms independent of PTH and mineral metabolism. Retrospective analyses of data from dialysis patients revealed increased survival with treatment with vitamin D analogs in the order of paricalcitol = doxercalciferol > calcitriol > no analog therapy [55-57]. Consistent with the survival data, patients treated with paricalcitol or doxercalciferol had fewer hospitalizations and hospital days per year than those treated with calcitriol [58, 59]. A detailed review of the survival data is presented in Chapter 7.

A major effort is underway to elucidate the mechanism(s) responsible for the greater survival with vitamin D analog therapy. The vitamin D receptor is widely distributed and active vitamin D compounds can affect a multitude of biological processes that could contribute to the increased survival. The focus of the research has been on actions of vitamin D analogs that may prevent progression of renal failure, inflammation and cardiovascular disease, the primary cause of death in CKD patients.

The renin-angiotensin system (RAS), *via* its active product angiotensin II (Ang II), exerts pathological effects in the cardiovascular system and the kidney [60, 61]. Renin converts angiotensinogen to Ang I which is converted by the angiotensin converting enzyme (ACE) to Ang II. ACE inhibitors and Ang II receptor blockers can slow progression of renal disease and proteinuria [62, 63], but ACE inhibitors also lead to increases in renin, which can exert its own deleterious effects. Vitamin D receptor activation inhibits renin gene transcription [64], decreasing the effects of both Ang II and renin.

The renoprotective effects of vitamin D analogs has been demonstrated in several animal models [65]. Paricalcitol treatment of mice with obstructive nephropathy (unilateral ureteral obstruction) attenuated the interstitial fibrosis [66]. Similarly, the glomerulosclerosis in rats injected with anti-thy-1.1 antibodies was reduced by treatment with maxacalcitol [67]. In uremic rats, paricalcitol suppressed the renal RAS and reduced tubulointerstitial and glomerular damage and lowered blood pressure [68]. Combined therapy with vitamin D analogs and ACE inhibitors has been shown to be effective. Studies in uremic rats demonstrated that paricalcitol, alone or with the ACE inhibitor enalopril, reduced renal fibrosis and inflammation [69] and cardiac oxidative stress [70]. Similar renoprotective effects of paricalcitol and doxercalciferol, combined with Ang II receptor blocker losartin, were reported in the streptozotocin-induced mouse model of diabetic nephropathy [71, 72]. In patients, paricalcitol reduced inflammation (lower serum C-reactive protein) and decreased albuminuria, with no changes in blood pressure or serum PTH at the doses used [73].

Active vitamin D compounds can potentially worsen the vascular calcification associated with CKD, especially at high doses that stimulate profound calcium absorption. However, several studies in animal models of CKD have reported that paricalcitol induces less calcification than doxercalciferol and calcitriol [31, 33, 74, 75], and it was demonstrated that lower doses of paricalcitol may protect against calcification [76]. *In vitro* studies examining the effects of vitamin D compounds on calcification of vascular smooth muscle cells produced mixed results [31, 74].

CANCER: MECHANISMS FOR THE ANTI-TUMOR ACTIVITY OF VITAMIN D ANALOGS

There are substantial epidemiological data associating reduced sunlight exposure with the development of cancers of the colon, prostate, ovary, breast and many other tissues [77-79], suggesting a role for vitamin D insufficiency in their development. However, most of the studies did not measure vitamin D levels, and little causal evidence is available.

The antiproliferative and differentiating activities of calcitriol and its analogs were first demonstrated in melanoma [80] and myeloid leukemia [81] cells. Since the VDR is present in most cell types and in tumors arsing from them, there is considerable interest in using vitamin D compounds to block tumor progression. As for other diseases, the use of calcitriol is limited by its potent calcemic activity, and, therefore, less calcemic analogs have been tested for their potential in treating several types of cancer, as discussed below.

The mechanisms by which vitamin D compounds can control cell growth are complex and can be cell-specific. Fig **3** summarizes some of the many documented means by which calcitriol and its analogs can control cell proliferation. Perhaps the most common pathway leads to the cyclin/CDK-mediated phosphorylation of the pocket proteins, retinoblastoma (Rb), p107 and p130. Hypophosphorylated pocket proteins bind to the E2F transcription factors and prevent their activation of DNA replication genes [82]. Calcitriol reduces the expression of cyclins D1, D3, E and A, and increases the cyclin-dependent kinase inhibitors p19, p21 and p27. These actions are complex and involve transcriptional and post-transcriptional mechanisms. Calcitriol can also alter many factors that act upstream of the cyclin/CDK system (*e.g.* Egr-1, TGFβ, IGFBP3 and the EGFR pathway), often in a cell-specific manner. For additional details of vitamin D-mediated growth inhibition and comprehensive references, the readers are directed to several excellent recent reviews [83-85].

The anti-cancer actions of calcitriol can also involve apoptosis, anti-angiogenesis and autophagy. Repression of the anti-apoptotic, pro-survival proteins Bcl-2 and Bcl-X or inducing the pro-apoptotic proteins BAX, BAK and BAD (reviewed in [84]) can lead to programmed cell death. The mechanisms can be cell-specific, and may be caspase-dependent or independent. Apoptosis may also involve destabilization of telomerase reverse transcriptase (TERT) mRNA, leading to telomere attrition and cell senescence [86]. Calcitriol may also halt tumor growth by blocking angiogenesis and endothelial cells growth [87, 88]. Calcitriol can induce autophagic cell death in breast cancer cells *in vitro* [89, 90], and the Gemini-23-yne-26,27-F6-1,25$(OH)_2D_3$ analog was found to inhibit AKT/mTOR signaling leading to a block in protein synthesis and cell growth arrest [91]. Vitamin D compounds can also repress the expression of Cox2, which could play a role in the control of various cancers, including prostate [92] and colon [93]. Most recently, one vitamin D analog, 1,25$(OH)_2$-16-ene-23-yne-D_3, was found to be selective, direct inhibitor of Cox-2 enzyme activity [94].

CANCER: PRE-CLINICAL STUDIES AND CLINICAL TRIALS

While much of our understanding of the anti-tumor potential of calcitriol and its analogs was derived through studies with normal and tumor-derived cell lines, the current article will focus mainly on *in vivo* testing. While hypercalcemia could be considered a relatively minor side effect of calcitriol in comparison to those for other chemotherapeutic drugs, the ideal would be to utilize analogs with less calcemic activity and greater specificity for the prevention, arrest, and cure of cancer. Clinical trials have been performed or in progress for a number of vitamain D analogs. Readers are directed to ClinicalTrials.gov for the current status of these trials.

Leukemia

Calcitriol is a potent modulator of hematopoiesis. In fact, the ability of calcitriol to promote differentiation and block proliferation of murine myeloid leukemia cells *in vitro* was one of the first nonclassical actions of the vitamin D hormone to be recognized [81]. Preclinical studies demonstrated prolonged survival of mice injected with leukemic cell line by calcitriol or 1α$(OH)D_3$ with the latter producing greater survival time at doses that did not cause hypercalcemia [95], and with the less calcemic analogs, 1,25$(OH)_2$-16-ene-23-yne-D_3 and 1,25$(OH)_2$-16-ene-5,6-trans-D_3 [96, 97]. Clinical trials with calcitriol for treatment of acute myelogenous leukemia revealed no beneficial effects and most patients became hypercalcemic [98, 99]. Similar disappointing results were obtained with 1α$(OH)D_3$ [100, 101], and in initial trials with paricalcitol [102]. Currently, there are ongoing clinical trials testing the efficacies of calcitriol, paricalcitol and doxercalciferol in treating myelodysplastic syndrome (see http://www.clinicaltrials.gov).

Colon Cancer

The inhibition of tumor growth in mice bearing human colon cancer (COLO 206F) cells was the first indication that vitamin D compounds could block solid tumor growth *in vivo* [103]. Similar anti-tumor effects in mice bearing colon cancer cells were demonstrated for 22(S)-24-homo-26,27-hexafluoro-1,22,25$(OH)_3D_3$ [104], EB1089 (1,25-dihydroxy-22, 24-diene-24,26,27-trishomo-D_3) (see Chapter 5), [105], paricalcitol [106], and Gemini, an analog of calcitriol with two side chains, and its hexadeuterated form (Fig. **1**) [107]. The analogs 1,25$(OH)_2$-16-ene-23-yne-26,27-hexafluoro-D_3 [108], 1α$(OH)D_5$ (1α(OH)-24-ethyl-D_3) [109] and maxacalcitol [110] were found to block carcinogen-induce colonic tumor growth. Successful tumor suppression was achieved with mild or no increases in serum calcium. Clinical trials beyond phase I for colon cancer have not been initiated.

Breast Cancer

The first demonstration of the potential of vitamin D therapy for breast cancer was the growth-inhibition of ER-negative MX-1 human breast cancer cells in athymic mice by maxacalcitol [111]; the effects were synergistic with those of adriamycin [111] and tamoxifen [112]. Maxacalcitol also inhibited growth of rat mammary tumors induced by 7,12-dimethybenz[a]anthracene with no effect on calcium [113].

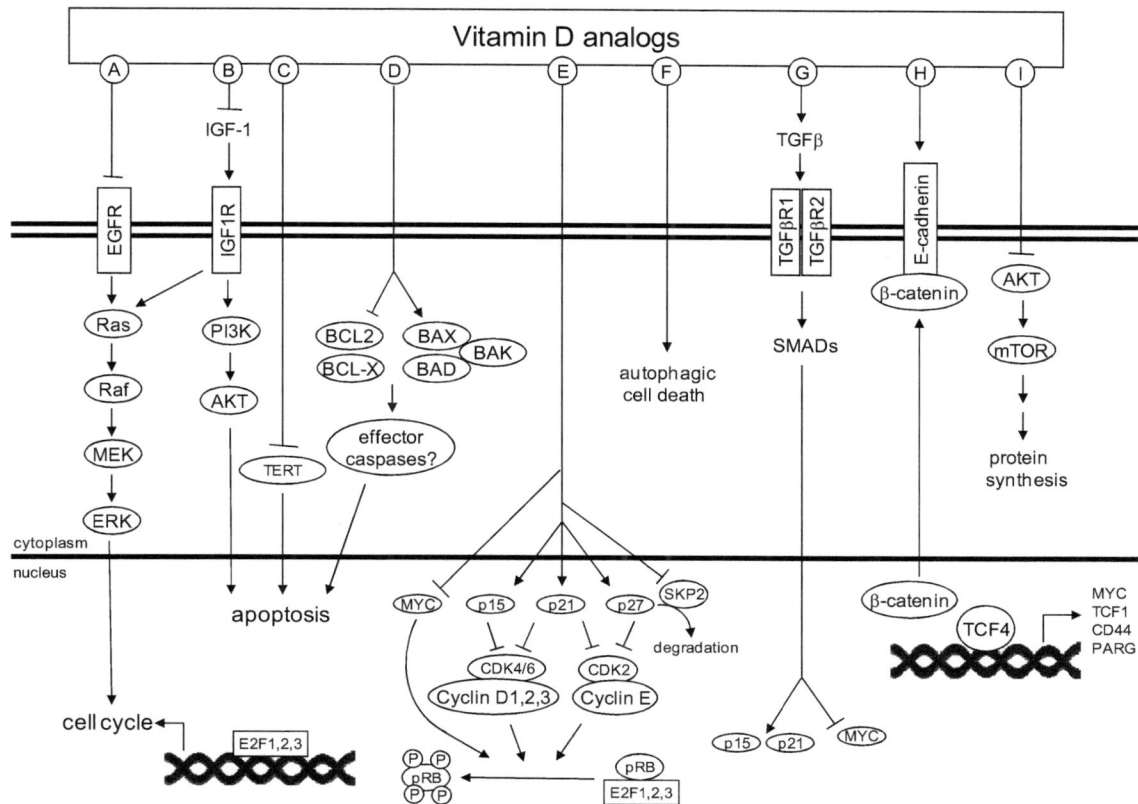

Figure 3: Mechanisms for the anti-proliferative actions of vitamin D compounds. Vitamin D compounds can regulate cell proliferation through many pathways. A. Suppression of epidermal growth factor receptor (EGFR) blocks downstream signaling through the pro-proliferative Ras/Raf/MEK/ERK1/2 MAP kinase pathway. B. Decreasing IGF-1 also reduces both ERK1/2 signaling and the pro-survival PI3K/Akt pathway, leading to apoptosis. C. Destabilization of the mRNA for telomerase reverse transcriptase (TERT) leads to telomerase attrition and cell death. D. Induction of the pro-apoptotic BAX, BAK and BAD and suppression of the anti-apoptotic BCL-2 and BCL-X leads to cell death. The apoptosis may be dependent or independent of effector caspases. E. Direct induction of the cyclin-dependent kinase inhibitors p15, p21 and p27 or suppression of cMyc can block cyclindependent phosphorylation of the pocket proteins pRB, p107 and p130, preventing the release of the proproliferative E2F transcription factors. In addition, vitamin D compounds can suppress the expression of cyclins D1, D2, D3 and E (not shown). F. In some cells, vitamin D analogs can promote autophagic cell death; details of the mechanism are under investigation. G. Increasing p15 and p21 and suppressing cMyc can be mediated indirectly by the TGFβ pathway. H. Induction of E-cadherin anchors -catenin to the membrane-associated cytoskeleton and prevents β-catenin from dimerizing with TCF4 to activate pro-proliferative genes. I. A Gemini analog was found to inhibit the Akt/mTOR pathway, thereby reducing the translation of growth promoting gene products.

In rats bearing mammary tumors induced by nitrosomethylurea (NMU), $1\alpha(OH)D_3$ [114], EB1089 [115], $1\alpha(OH)D_5$ [116], and $1\alpha,25$-dihydroxy-16-ene-23-yne-26,27-hexafluoro-vitamin D_3 [117] were all shown to be effective in reducing tumor growth, with the last acting synergistically with tamoxifen [117]. Growth of tumors of MCF-7 breast cancer cells injected into athymic mice was reduced by 75% with EB1089 treatment and was associated with induction of markers of apoptosis [118], suggesting that vitamin D compounds may be able to regress existing tumors in addition to slowing their growth. Importantly, the analogs can act synergistically with other treatments as shown for maxacalcitol (with adriamycin [111] and tamoxifen [112]) and $1\alpha,25$-dihydroxy-16-ene-23-yne-26,27-hexafluoro-vitamin D_3 (with paclitaxel [119]. In addition, the calcemic effects can be reduced by co-treatment with bisphosphonates, as in a study demonstrating the efficacy of $1,24(OH)_2D_3$ and calcitriol in reducing tumor growth in mice injected with 16/C mouse mammary adrenocarcinoma cells [120].

In a small trial with 14 breast cancer patients, topical application of calcipotriol (100 μg daily) produced modest response (50% reduction in lesion diameter) in three patients and a lesser response in another [121]. Additional trials have not been reported.

Prostate Cancer

Prostate cancer is the most commonly diagnosed malignancy in U.S. males. Extensive *in vitro* studies of the effect of calcitriol on growth of prostatic cell lines and primary cultures of prostate tumors suggested that prostate cancer could be a target for vitamin D therapy [122]. Suppression of prostate growth by vitamin D compounds may involve inhibition of Cox2 and its prostaglandin products [123], blocking autophosphorylation of the receptors for KGF and IGF-1, and reducing bcl-2 [124].

Preclinical studies in mice inoculated with prostate cell lines LNCaP or PC-3, found that calcitriol treatment reduced tumor weight [125], while others found that calcitriol and $1,25(OH)_2$-16-ene-23-yne-D_3 slowed the growth of PC-3 cells in mice [126]. In a rat model of prostate cancer, prophylactic $1,25(OH)_2$-16-ene-23-yne-26,27-hexafluoro-vitamin D_3 treatment decreased tumor incidence by over 40% [127]. Growth reduction of prostate cells *in vivo* was also achieved with the vitamin D analogs EB1089 [128] and maxacalcitol, which are less calcemic than calcitriol.

Metastasis of prostate cancer may also be reduced by vitamin D analogs. 1α-hydroxymethyl-16-ene-26,27-bishomo-25-hydroxy-D_3 reduced the occurrance of bone lesions in SCID mice injected with the MDA-PCa 2b prostate cancer line (30% of mice *vs.* 90% in vehicle controls). There were no incidents of hypercalcemia, despite the presence of tumor cells in 70% of the analog-treated mice. Studies *in vitro* indicated that the analog prevented a mitogenic response of osteoblasts to growth factors released by the tumor cells.

In relation to prostate cancer, the analog 1α-fluoro-25-hydroxy-16,23E-diene-26,27-bishomo-20-epi-D_3 (BXL-628) was found to reduce prostate cell proliferation and induce apoptosis in intact and testosterone-treated rats to an extent equivalent to finasteride [124], and without increasing serum calcium. Phase II studies confirmed the effectiveness of BXL-628 in arresting prostate growth in patients with benign prostatic hyperplasia [129]. However, as discussed in Chapter 5, all further clinical development of BXL-628 has been terminated.

In a small clinical trial, calcitriol therapy had no effect on tumor mass in 11 patients with hormone-refractory metastatic prostate cancer, even at doses that produced hypercalcemia [130]. However, in another study in patients with androgen-independent prostate cancer, combination therapy with high dose calcitriol and docetaxel produced a slight increase in survival compared to docetaxel alone (24.5 *vs.* 16.4 months) [131]. See ClinicalTrials.gov for updates on the trials for prostate cancer.

Pancreatic Cancer

The antiproliferative effects of calcitriol and maxacalcitol agents on tumor size of xenografts of pancreatic cell lines inoculated into athymic mice has been studied [132]. Both compounds inhibited proliferation in 3 of 9 cell lines *in vitro*. However, *in vivo,* maxacalcitol suppressed proliferation of BxPC-3 xenografts more significantly than calcitriol, without induction of hypercalcemia. In another study, paricalcitol inhibited pancreatic cell growth *in vitro* and *in vivo* in mice without hypercalcemia, and suppression of tumor growth was accompanied by induction of p21 and p27 [133]. Pancreatic cancer cells can also produce calcitriol and are growth-inhibited by exogenous $25(OH)D_3$ [134], suggesting that adequate vitamin D status may slow tumor growth.

Skin Cancer

Epidemiological data supports a role for vitamin D status in susceptibility to various types of cancer, and suggests a protective role for endogenous production of vitamin D_3 by sun exposure and D. While excessive UV irradiation can cause skin cancers, recent data indicate a protective effect of vitamin D compounds against skin cancer as well. Topical application of calcitriol and analogs prior to ultra violet radiation reduced immunosuppression and DNA damage in mice [135].

Other Cancers

Neuroblastoma, a pediatric tumor derived from neuroectodermal cells and the most common extracranial solid tumor in childhood, has been treated successfully in xenograft models with the vitamin D analogs 1-

hydroxymethyl-16-ene-24, 24-F$_2$-26, 27-bishomo-25-(OH)D$_3$ and EB1089 [136] and with doxercalciferol [137]. 1,25(OH)$_2$-16-ene-23-yne-vitamin D$_3$ and doxercalciferol were shown to reduce tumor growth in mouse models of retinoblastoma, but the effective doses caused substantial, even toxic, hypercalcemia [138].

In a xenograft model for ovarian cancer in mice, the analog EB1089 reduced tumor growth at doses that were not hypercalcemic [139] by stabilizing p27, increasing GADD45 and inducing apoptosis *via* destabilization of telomerase catalytic subunit mRNA [140]. No clinical trials have been reported for treatment of ovarian cancer with vitamin D analogs.

Treatment of lung cancer has also been investigated. Maxacalcitol, at non-calcemic doses, inhibited metastasis and angiogenesis in mice implanted with the Lewis lung carcinoma [141]. Curiously, the efficacy was retained in VDR-ablated mice. A clinical trial for calcitriol in the treatment of non-small cell lung cancer is underway.

IMMUNOMODULATORY ACTIONS OF VITAMIN D

Calcitriol has emerged as an important modulator of immune function. Most cells of the immune system, including antigen-presenting cells (macrophages and dendritic cells), and activated B and T lymphocytes, express the VDR. Calcitriol prevents Th1 cell development and release of IL-2 and IFN-γ, while enhancing development of the tolerogenic Th2 cells. The native vitamin D hormone induces dendritic cells to acquire tolerogenic properties that lead to induction of regulatory rather than effector T cells. In addition, VDR activation reduces the expression of the costimulatory molecules CD40, CD80 and CD86, as well as IL-12 and enhances the expression of IL-10. Together, these actions lead to an overall immunosuppression, suggesting beneficial potential of calcitriol and its analogs for the treatment of autoimmune diseases and transplantation. B cell-related disorders, including lupus erythematosus, may also be targets of vitamin D therapy, since activation of the VDR in B lymphocytes inhibits proliferation and immunoglobulin production [142].

There is evidence for autocrine regulation of the immune system by vitamin D. Many cells, including macrophages, dendritic cells and T cells, express the 1α-hydroxylase (CYP27B1). For example, activation of macrophages through Toll-like receptors induces expression of the CYP27B1 and the VDR [143], facilitating the activation of 25(OH)D$_3$ to calcitriol which, in turn, induces the antimicrobial peptide, cathelicidin.

Fig. **4** illustrates the immunomodulatory actions of vitamin D compounds. Further details on the role of vitamin D in the immune system and potential therapeutic applications can be found in several recent reviews [129, 144-146].

Autoimmune Diseases

Type I diabetes may be a target for vitamin D therapy. Studies in a mouse model (non-obese diabetic or NOD mice) that spontaneously develops insulitis showed that calcitriol can prevent development of diabetes if administered before the onset of insulitis at 3 weeks of age. This model has been used to identify a number of less calcemic analogs that may be therapeutically useful, KH1060 (Fig. **1**) [147], 1,25(OH)$_2$-16,23-diene-26,27-F$_6$-19-nor-D$_3$ [148], and 19-nor-14,20-bis-epi-23-yne-1,25(OH)$_2$D$_3$ [149].

Experimental allergic encephalomyelitis (EAE), produced by inoculation of mice with myelin basic protein, is used as a model for multiple sclerosis, since Th1-type cells specific for myelin antigens underlie both diseases. Induction of EAE can be prevented by calcitriol [150, 151] and the less calcemic analogs, 1,25(OH)$_2$-24-bishomo-23,24-diene-D$_3$ [152] and 19-nor-14,20-bisepi-23-yne-1,25(OH)$_2$D$_3$ [153]. Calcitriol and its 20-epi analog can inhibit the progression of arthritis in a rodent model produced by immunization with collagen type II [154, 155].

Lupus and other autoimmune disorders in the MRL mouse model can be prevented by calcitriol [156], 1,24(OH)$_2$D$_3$ [157] and maxacalcitol [158]. The anti-inflammatory actions of calcitriol were found to block progression and reduce symptoms in the IL-10-ablated mouse model of inflammatory bowel disease [159].

At present, no studies using selective analogs have been reported, but those capable of preventing or ameliorating other autoimmune disease would be likely candidates.

Transplantation

In experimental animals, survival of allografts of aorta, bone, bone marrow, heart, kidney, liver, pancreatic islets, skin and small intestine were significantly prolonged by administration of various vitamin D compounds (reviewed in [144]). Furthermore, at least two studies found enhanced allograft survival with a combination of vitamin D analogs (KH1060 and MC1288) and cyclosporin A [160, 161]. The use of vitamin D analogs for immunosuppression may allow lower, less toxic doses of cyclosporin A to be administered, and may provide alternatives to glucocorticoids in combined therapeutic regimens.

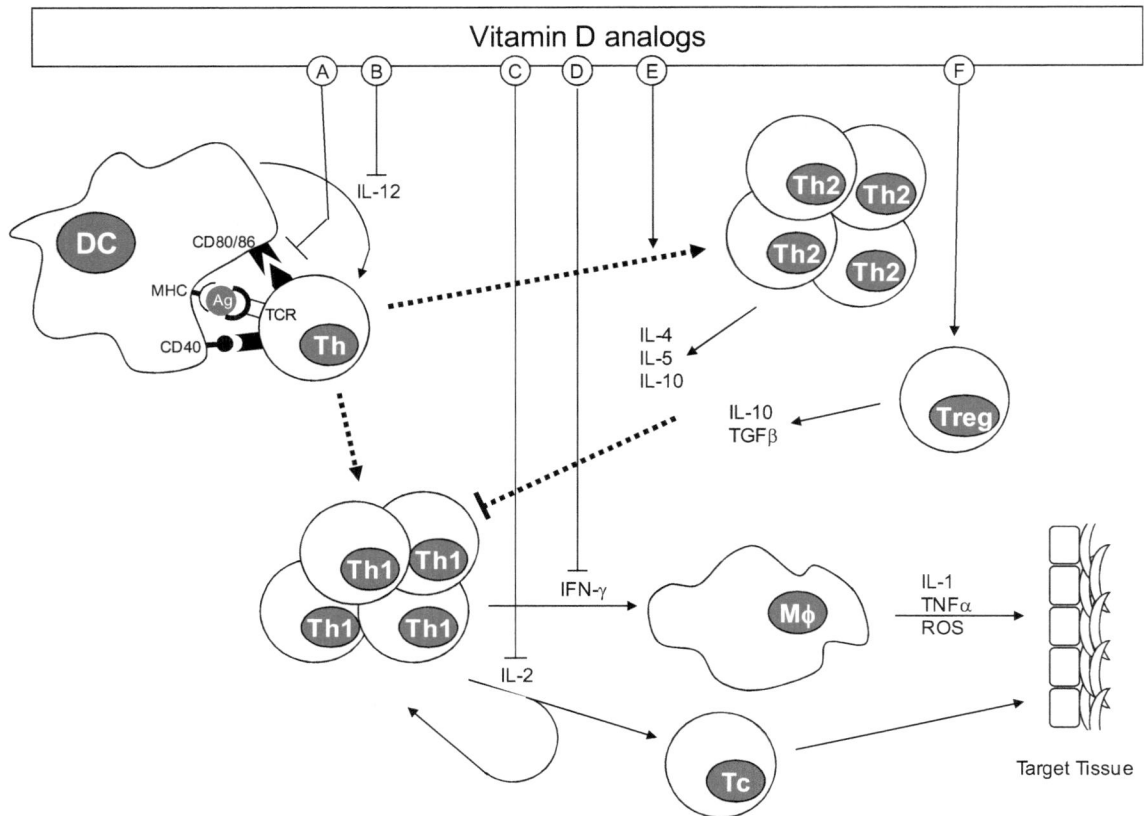

Figure 4: The immunomodulatory actions of vitamin D compounds. Vitamin D compounds exert multiple actions on various factors leading to a reduction in pro-inflammatory Th1 cells in favor of the more regulatory Th2 cells. (A) Reduction in MHC II-complexed antigen (Ag) and co-stimulatory molecules (CD40, 80 and 86) on dendritic cells as well as inhibition of IL-12 (B), shifting the T helper cells (Th) conversion from the Th1 to the Th2 phenotype. (C) Suppression of IL-2 by Th1 cells disrupts the positive feedback loop for Th1 proliferation and activation cytotoxic T cells (Tc). (D) Blocking IFN-γ reduces macrophage activation. (E) Vitamin D compounds promote the proliferation of Th2 cells and (F) the formation of regulatory T cells (Treg) which are immunosuppressive. Cytokines released by the Th2 and Treg cells in response to vitamin D compounds further suppress Th1 proliferation.

OSTEOPOROSIS

Osteoporosis is a disorder of bone metabolism characterized by an uncoupling of bone resorption and bone formation, with a net loss of bone mass and susceptibility to fractures. Active vitamin D compounds can regulate both aspects of bone turnover through direct and indirect mechanisms, and therefore a potential role for calcitriol and its analogs has been sought. Studies with calcitriol or its synthetic precursor, alfacalcidol, found increases in bone mineral density [162-168], due in part to enhanced calcium absorption. Decreased bone fracture rate was observed in some [165-168], but not all, studies. Combined treatment of alfacalcidol with the bisphosphonate alendronate enhanced bone mass with fewer falls and fractures [169].

The vitamin D analog ED-71 ($1,25(OH)_2$-2β(3-hydroxypropoxy)-vitamin D_3 (see Fig. **1**) was shown to increase bone mass in ovariectomized rats [170] and to counteract glucocorticoid-induced osteopenia by increasing intestinal calcium absorption, reducing bone resorption, and enhancing bone mineralization [171]. Studies in patients confirmed its effectiveness in maintaining bone mass in post-menopausal osteoporosis [172]. ED-71 (eldecalcitol) has now been approved for treatment of osteoporosi in Japan.

The analog 2MD (2-Methylene-19-nor-20-epi-$1,25(OH)_2D_3$) which is also modified at carbon 2, was also effective in preventing the decrease in bone density in ovariectomized rats, primarily by enhancing bone formation, but with little inhibitory action on bone resorption [173-175]. However, clinical trials for this analog have been discontinued.

DISCUSSION/CONCLUSION

Calcitriol and its analogs have tremendous potential for the treatment of cancer, psoriasis, hyperparathyroidism, autoimmune diseases, and osteoporosis. Use of calcitriol, in most cases, is limited by its high calcemic activity. However, newer analogs have been developed that have greater selectivity for various target cells, but lower calcemic and phosphatemic activities. Analogs for psoriasis (calcipotriol) and for hyperparathyroidism (paricalcitol, doxercalciferol, maxacalcitol and falecalcitriol) are currently in use and others are in development and undergoing clinical trials. The molecular basis for the selectivity of the most of the analogs is under investigation [176]. A better understanding of the mechanisms may allow the development of even more effective vitamin D analogs.

DISCLOSURE

Part of the information in this chapter has been previously published: Brown and Slatopolsky, Molecular Aspects of Medicine, Volume 29, Issue 6, Pages 433-452, December 2008.

REFERENCES

[1]   Dusso AS, Brown AJ, Slatopolsky E: Vitamin D. Am J Physiol Renal Physiol 2005; 289(1): F8-28.

[2]   Kragballe K, Wildfang IL: Calcipotriol (MC 903), a novel vitamin D3 analogue stimulates terminal differentiation and inhibits proliferation of cultured human keratinocytes. Archives of Dermatological Research 1990; 282(3): 164-7.

[3]   Zhang JZ, Maruyama K, Ono I, Iwatsuki K, Kaneko F: Regulatory effects of 1,25-dihydroxyvitamin D3 and a novel vitamin D3 analogue MC903 on secretion of interleukin-1 alpha (IL-1 alpha) and IL-8 by normal human keratinocytes and a human squamous cell carcinoma cell line (HSC-1). Journal of Dermatological Science 1994; 7(1): 24-31.

[4]   Maruyama K, Zhang JZ, Nihei Y, Ono I, Kaneko F: Regulatory effects of antipsoriatic agents on interleukin-1 alpha production by human keratinocytes stimulated with gamma interferon *in vitro*. Skin Pharmacology 1995; 8(1-2): 41-8.

[5]   Binderup L, Bramm E: Effects of a novel vitamin D analogue MC903 on cell proliferation and differentiation *in vitro* and on calcium metabolism *in vivo*. Biochemical Pharmacology 1988; 37(5): 889-95.

[6]   Binderup L: Immunological properties of vitamin D analogues and metabolites. Biochemical Pharmacology 1992; 43(9): 1885-92.

[7]   Nishimura M, Makino Y, Matugi H: Tacalcitol ointment for psoriasis. Acta Dermato-Venereologica. Supplementum 1994; 186: 166-8.

[8]   Matsunaga T, Yamamoto M, Mimura H, *et al.*: 1,24(R)-dihydroxyvitamin D3, a novel active form of vitamin D3 with high activity for inducing epidermal differentiation but decreased hypercalcemic activity. Journal of Dermatology 1990; 17(3): 135-42.

[9]   Morimoto S, Imanaka S, Koh E, *et al.*: Comparison of the inhibitions of proliferation of normal and psoriatic fibroblasts by 1 alpha,25-dihydroxyvitamin D3 and synthetic analogues of vitamin D3 with an oxygen atom in their side chain. Biochemistry International 1989; 19(5): 1143-9.

[10]   Barker JN, Ashton RE, Marks R, Harris RI, Berth-Jones J: Topical maxacalcitol for the treatment of psoriasis vulgaris: a placebo-controlled, double-blind, dose-finding study with active comparator. Br J Dermatol 1999; 141(2): 274-8.

[11]   Slatopolsky E, Brown AJ, Dusso A: Pathogenesis of secondary hyperparathyroidism. Kidney International 1999; 73: S14-9.

[12]   Pande S, Ritter CS, Rothstein M, *et al.*: FGF-23 and sFRP-4 in chronic kidney disease and post-renal transplantation. Nephron Physiol 2006; 104(1): p23-32.

[13]   Hruska KA, Saab G, Mathew S, Lund R: Renal osteodystrophy, phosphate homeostasis, and vascular calcification. Semin Dial 2007; 20(4): 309-15.

[14]   Brown AJ, Slatopolsky E: Drug insight: vitamin D analogs in the treatment of secondary hyperparathyroidism in patients with chronic kidney disease. Nat Clin Pract Endocrinol Metab 2007; 3(2): 134-44.

[15]   Brown AJ, Ritter CR, Finch JL, *et al.*: The noncalcemic analogue of vitamin D, 22-oxacalcitriol, suppresses parathyroid hormone synthesis and secretion. Journal of Clinical Investigation 1989; 84(3): 728-32.

[16]   Murayama E, Miyamoto K, Kubodera N, Mori T, Matsunaga I: Synthetic studies of vitamin D3 analogues. VIII. Synthesis of 22-oxavitamin D3 analogues. Chemical & Pharmaceutical Bulletin 1986; 34(10): 4410-3.

[17]   Brown AJ, Finch JL, Lopez-Hilker S, *et al.*: New active analogues of vitamin D with low calcemic activity. Kidney International 1990; 29 (suppl 29): S22-7.

[18]   Naveh-Many T, Silver J: Effects of calcitriol, 22-oxacalcitriol, and calcipotriol on serum calcium and parathyroid hormone gene expression. Endocrinology 1993; 133(6): 2724-8.

[19]   Hirata M, Endo K, Katsumata K, Ichikawa F, Kubodera N, Fukagawa M: A comparison between 1,25-dihydroxy-22-oxavitamin D3 and 1,25-dihydroxyvitamin D3 regarding suppression of parathyroid hormone and calcemic action. Nephology, Dialysis Transplantation 2002; 17(suppl 10): 41-5.

[20]   Monier-Faugere MC, Geng Z, Friedler RM, *et al.*: 22-oxacalcitriol suppresses secondary hyperparathyroidism without inducing low bone turnover in dogs with renal failure. Kidney International 1999; 55(3): 821-32.

[21]   Hirata M, Katsumata K, Masaki T, *et al.*: 22-Oxacalcitriol ameliorates high-turnover bone and marked osteitis fibrosa in rats with slowly progressive nephritis. Kidney International 1999; 56: 2040-2047.

[22]   Tamura S, Ueki K, Mashimo K, *et al.*: Comparison of the efficacy of an oral calcitriol pulse or intravenous 22-oxacalcitriol therapies in chronic hemodialysis patients. Clin Exp Nephrol 2005; 9(3): 238-43.

[23]   Akizawa T, Kurokawa K: [Long-term clinical effect of maxacalcitol on hemodialysis patients with secondary hyperparathyroidism]. Clin Calcium 2002; 12(6): 781-8.

[24]   Akizawa T, Ohashi Y, Akiba T, *et al.*: Dose-response study of 22-oxacalcitriol in patients with secondary hyperparathyroidism. Ther Apher Dial 2004; 8(6): 480-91.

[25]   Yasuda M, Akiba T, Nihei H: Multicenter clinical trial of 22-oxa-1,25-dihydroxyvitamin D3 for chronic dialysis patients. Am J Kidney Dis 2003; 41(3 Suppl 1): S108-11.

[26]   Hayashi M, Tsuchiya Y, Itaya Y, *et al.*: Comparison of the effects of calcitriol and maxacalcitol on secondary hyperparathyroidism in patients on chronic haemodialysis: a randomized prospective multicentre trial. Nephrol Dial Transplant 2004; 19(8): 2067-73.

[27]   Akizawa T, Suzuki M, Akiba T, *et al.*: Long-term effect of 1,25-dihydroxy-22-oxavitamin D(3) on secondary hyperparathyroidism in haemodialysis patients. One-year administration study. Nephrol Dial Transplant 2002; 17 Suppl 10: 28-36.

[28]   Slatopolsky E, Finch J, Ritter C, *et al.*: A new analog of calcitriol, 19-nor-1,25-(OH)2D2, suppresses parathyroid hormone secretion in uremic rats in the absence of hypercalcemia. American Journal of Kidney Diseases 1995; 26(5): 852-60.

[29]   Takahashi F, Finch JL, Denda M, Dusso AS, Brown AJ, Slatopolsky E: A new analog of 1,25-(OH)2D3, 19-nor-1,25-(OH)2D2, suppresses serum PTH and parathyroid gland growth in uremic rats without elevation of intestinal vitamin D receptor content. American Journal of Kidney Diseases 1997; 30(1): 105-12.

[30]   Slatopolsky E, Cozzolino M, Lu Y, *et al.*: Efficacy of 19-Nor-1,25-(OH)2D2 in the prevention and treatment of hyperparathyroid bone disease in experimental uremia. Kidney Int 2003; 63(6): 2020-7.

[31]   Cardus A, Panizo S, Parisi E, Fernandez E, Valdivielso JM: Differential effects of vitamin D analogs on vascular calcification. Journal of Bone and Mineral Research 2007; 22(6): 860-6.

[32]   Wu-Wong JR, Nakane M, Ma J, Ruan X, Kroeger PE: Effects of Vitamin D analogs on gene expression profiling in human coronary artery smooth muscle cells. Atherosclerosis 2006; 186(1): 20-8.

[33]   Mizobuchi M, Finch JL, Martin DR, Slatopolsky E: Differential effects of vitamin D receptor activators on vascular calcification in uremic rats. Kidney International 2007; 72(6): 709-15.

[34]   Martin KJ, Gonzales EA, Gellens M, Hamm LL, Abboud H, Lindberg J: 19-Nor-1a,25-dihydroxyvitamin D2 (Paricalcitol) safely and effectively reduces the levels of intact parathyroid hormone in patients on hemodialysis. Journal of the American Society of Nephrology 1998; 9: 1427-32.

[35]   Martin KJ, Gonzalez EA, Gellens ME, Hamm LL, Abboud H, Lindberg J: Therapy of secondary hyperparathyroidism with 19-nor-1a,25-dihydroxyvitamin D2. American Journal of Kidney Diseases 1998; 32: S 61-S 66.

[36]   Sprague SM, Llach F, Amdahl M, Taccetta C, Batlle D: Paricalcitol versus calcitriol in the treatment of secondary hyperparathyroidism. Kidney Int 2003; 63(4): 1483-90.

[37]   Sjoden G, Smith C, Lindgren U, DeLuca HF: 1a-Hydroxyvitamin D2 is less toxic than 1a-hydroxyvitamin D3 in the rat. Proceedings of the Society for Experimental Biology & Medicine 1985; 178(3): 432-6.

[38]   Tan AU, Levine BS, Mazess Rb, et al.: Effective suppression of parathyroid hormone by 1a-hydroxy-vitamin D2 in hemodialysis patients with moderate to severe secondary hyperparathyroidism. Kidney International 1997; 51(1): 317-23.

[39]   Frazao JM, Chesney RW, Coburn JW: Intermittent oral 1ahydroxyvitamin D2 is effective and safe for the suppression of secondary hyperparathyroidism in haemodialysis patients. Nephrology, Dialysis, Transplantation 1998; 3: 68-72.

[40]   Coburn JW, Maung HM, Elangovan L, et al.: Doxercalciferol safely suppresses PTH levels in patients with secondary hyperparathyroidism associated with chronic kidney disease stages 3 and 4. Am J Kidney Dis 2004; 43(5): 877-90.

[41]   Slatopolsky E, Cozzolino M, Finch JL: Differential effects of 19-nor-1,25-(OH)(2)D(2) and 1alpha-hydroxyvitamin D(2) on calcium and phosphorus in normal and uremic rats. Kidney Int 2002; 62(4): 1277-84.

[42]   Zisman AL, Ghantous W, Schinleber P, Roberts L, Sprague SM: Inhibition of parathyroid hormone: a dose equivalency study of paricalcitol and doxercalciferol. Am J Nephrol 2005; 25(6): 591-5.

[43]   Joist HE, Ahya SN, Giles K, Norwood K, Slatopolsky E, Coyne DW: Differential effects of very high doses of doxercalciferol and paricalcitol on serum phosphorus in hemodialysis patients. Clin Nephrol 2006; 65(5): 335-41.

[44]   Hansen D, Brandi L, Rasmussen K: Treatment of secondary hyperparathyroidism in haemodialysis patients: a randomised clinical trial comparing paricalcitol and alfacalcidol. BMC Nephrol 2009; 10: 28.

[45]   Imanishi Y, Inaba M, Seki H, et al.: Increased biological potency of hexafluorinated analogs of 1,25-dihydroxyvitamin D3 on bovine parathyroid cells. J Steroid Biochem Mol Biol 1999; 70(4-6): 243-8.

[46]   Komuro S, Sato M, Kanamaru H: Disposition and metabolism of F6-1alpha,25(OH)2 vitamin D3 and 1alpha,25(OH)2 vitamin D3 in the parathyroid glands of rats dosed with tritium-labeled compounds. Drug Metab Dispos 2003; 31(8): 973-8.

[47]   Nishizawa Y, Morii H, Ogura Y, De Luca HF: Clinical trial of 26,26,26,27,27,27-hexafluoro-1,25-dihydroxyvitamin D3 in uremic patients on hemodialysis: preliminary report. Contributions to Nephrology 1991; 90: 196-203.

[48]   Ito H, Ogata H, Yamamoto M, et al.: Comparison of oral falecalcitriol and intravenous calcitriol in hemodialysis patients with secondary hyperparathyroidism: a randomized, crossover trial. Clinical Nephrology 2009; 71(6): 660-8.

[49]   Fan SLS, Schroeder NJ, Calverley MJ, Burrin JM, Makin HLJ, Cunningham J: Potent suppression of the parathyroid glands by hydroxylated metabolites of dihydrotachysterol(2). Nephology, Dialysis Transplantation 2000; 15: 1943-1949.

[50]   Hruby M, Urena P, Mannstadt M, Schmitt F, Lacour B, Drueke TB: Effects of new vitamin D analogues on parathyroid function in chronically uraemic rats with secondary hyperparathyroidism. Nephrology, Dialysis, Transplantation 1996; 11(9): 1781-6.

[51]   Lippuner K, Perrelet R, Casez JP, Popp A, Uskokovic MR, Jaeger P: 1,25-(OH)2-16ene-23yne-D3 reduces secondary hyperparathyroidism in uremic rats with little calcemic effect. Horm Res 2004; 61(1): 7-16.

[52]   Brown AJ, Ritter CS, Weiskopf AS, et al.: Isolation and identification of 1alpha-hydroxy-3-epi-vitamin D3, a potent suppressor of parathyroid hormone secretion. J Cell Biochem 2005; 96(3): 569-78.

[53]   Plum LA, Prahl JM, Ma X, et al.: Biologically active noncalcemic analogs of 1alpha,25-dihydroxyvitamin D with an abbreviated side chain containing no hydroxyl. Proc Natl Acad Sci U S A 2004; 101(18): 6900-4.

[54]   Slatopolsky E, Finch JL, Brown AJ, et al.: Effect of 2-methylene-19-nor-(20S)-1 alpha-hydroxy-bishomopregnacalciferol (2MbisP), an analog of vitamin D, on secondary hyperparathyroidism. Journal of Bone and Mineral Research 2007; 22(5): 686-94.

[55]   Teng M, Wolf M, Lowrie E, Ofsthun N, Lazarus M, Thadhani R: Survival of patients undergoing hemodialysis with paricalcitol or calcitriol therapy. New England Journal of Medicine 2003; 349: 446-456.

[56]   Teng M, Wolf M, Ofsthun MN, *et al.*: Activated injectable vitamin D and hemodialysis survival: a historical cohort study. J Am Soc Nephrol 2005; 16(4): 1115-25.

[57]   Tentori F, Hunt WC, Stidley CA, Rohrsceib MR, Meyer KB, Zager PG: Survival among hemodialysis patients receiving intravenous doxercalciferol and paricalcitol versus calcitriol. Journal of the American Society of Nephology 2005; 16: 279A.

[58]   Tentori F, Hunt WC, Rohrsceib MR, Stidley CA, Meyer KB, Zager PG: Decreased odds of hospitalization among hemodialysis patients receiving doxercalciferol and paricalcitol versus calcitriol. J Amer Soc Nephrol 2005; 16: 279A.

[59]   Dobrez DG, Mathes A, Amdahl M, Marx SE, Melnick JZ, Sprague SM: Paricalcitol-treated patients experience improved hospitalization outcomes compared with calcitriol-treated patients in real-world clinical settings. Nephrol Dial Transplant 2004; 19(5): 1174-81.

[60]   Brewster UC, Perazella MA: The renin-angiotensin-aldosterone system and the kidney: effects on kidney disease. American Journal of Medicine 2004; 116(4): 263-72.

[61]   Ruster C, Wolf G: Renin-angiotensin-aldosterone system and progression of renal disease. Journal of the American Society of Nephrology 2006; 17(11): 2985-91.

[62]   Andersen S, Tarnow L, Rossing P, Hansen BV, Parving HH: Renoprotective effects of angiotensin II receptor blockade in type 1 diabetic patients with diabetic nephropathy. Kidney International 2000; 57(2): 601-6.

[63]   Chan JC, Ko GT, Leung DH, *et al.*: Long-term effects of angiotensin-converting enzyme inhibition and metabolic control in hypertensive type 2 diabetic patients. Kidney International 2000; 57(2): 590-600.

[64]   Li YC, Qiao G, Uskokovic M, Xiang W, Zheng W, Kong J: Vitamin D: a negative endocrine regulator of the renin-angiotensin system and blood pressure. J Steroid Biochem Mol Biol 2004; 89-90(1-5): 387-92.

[65]   Li YC: Renoprotective effects of vitamin D analogs. Kidney International 2009.

[66]   Tan X, Li Y, Liu Y: Paricalcitol attenuates renal interstitial fibrosis in obstructive nephropathy. Journal of the American Society of Nephrology 2006; 17(12): 3382-93.

[67]   Makibayashi K, Tatematsu M, Hirata M, *et al.*: A vitamin D analog ameliorates glomerular injury on rat glomerulonephritis. American Journal of Pathology 2001; 158: 1733-41.

[68]   Freundlich M, Quiroz Y, Zhang Z, *et al.*: Suppression of renin-angiotensin gene expression in the kidney by paricalcitol. Kidney International 2008; 74(11): 1394-402.

[69]   Mizobuchi M, Morrissey J, Finch JL, *et al.*: Combination therapy with an angiotensin-converting enzyme inhibitor and a vitamin D analog suppresses the progression of renal insufficiency in uremic rats. Journal of the American Society of Nephrology 2007; 18(6): 1796-806.

[70]   Husain K, Ferder L, Mizobuchi M, Finch J, Slatopolsky E: Combination therapy with paricalcitol and enalapril ameliorates cardiac oxidative injury in uremic rats. American Journal of Nephrology 2009; 29(5): 465-72.

[71]   Zhang Z, Zhang Y, Ning G, Deb DK, Kong J, Li YC: Combination therapy with AT1 blocker and vitamin D analog markedly ameliorates diabetic nephropathy: blockade of compensatory renin increase. Proc Natl Acad Sci U S A 2008; 105(41): 15896-901.

[72]   Zhang Y, Deb DK, Kong J, *et al.*: Long-term therapeutic effect of vitamin D analog doxercalciferol on diabetic nephropathy: strong synergism with AT1 receptor antagonist. Am J Physiol Renal Physiol 2009; 297(3): F791-801.

[73]   Alborzi P, Patel NA, Peterson C, *et al.*: Paricalcitol reduces albuminuria and inflammation in chronic kidney disease: a randomized double-blind pilot trial. Hypertension 2008; 52(2): 249-55.

[74]   Wu-Wong JR, Noonan W, Ma J, *et al.*: Role of phosphorus and vitamin D analogs in the pathogenesis of vascular calcification. Journal of Pharmacology and Experimental Therapeutics 2006; 318(1): 90-8.

[75]   Wu-Wong JR, Melnick J: Vascular calcification in chronic kidney failure: role of vitamin D receptor. Curr Opin Investig Drugs 2007; 8(3): 237-47.

[76]   Mathew S, Lund RJ, Chaudhary LR, Geurs T, Hruska KA: Vitamin D receptor activators can protect against vascular calcification. Journal of the American Society of Nephrology 2008; 19(8): 1509-19.

[77]   Garland CF, Garland FC: Do sunlight and vitamin D reduce the likelihood of colon cancer? International Journal of Epidemiology 1980; 9(3): 227-31.

[78]   Garland FC, Garland CF, Gorham ED, Young JF: Geographic variation in breast cancer mortality in the United States: a hypothesis involving exposure to solar radiation. Preventive Medicine 1990; 19(6): 614-22.

[79]   Boscoe FP, Schymura MJ: Solar ultraviolet-B exposure and cancer incidence and mortality in the United States, 1993-2002. BMC Cancer 2006; 6: 264.

[80]   Colston K, Colston MJ, Feldman D: 1,25-dihydroxyvitamin D3 and malignant melanoma: the presence of receptors and inhibition of cell growth in culture. Endocrinology 1981; 108(3): 1083-6.

[81]   Abe E, Miyaura C, Sakagami H, *et al.*: Differentiation of mouse myeloid leukemia cells induced by 1 alpha,25-dihydroxyvitamin D3. Proceedings of the National Academy of Sciences of the United States of America 1981; 78(8): 4990-4.

[82]   Eelen G, Verlinden L, van Camp M, *et al.*: The effects of 1alpha,25-dihydroxyvitamin D3 on the expression of DNA replication genes. J Bone Miner Res 2004; 19(1): 133-46.

[83]   Eelen G, Gysemans C, Verlinden L, *et al.*: Mechanism and potential of the growth-inhibitory actions of vitamin D and ana-logs. Curr Med Chem 2007; 14(17): 1893-910.

[84]   Deeb KK, Trump DL, Johnson CS: Vitamin D signalling pathways in cancer: potential for anticancer therapeutics. Nat Rev Cancer 2007; 7(9): 684-700.

[85]   Ingraham BA, Bragdon B, Nohe A: Molecular basis of the potential of vitamin D to prevent cancer. Curr Med Res Opin 2008; 24(1): 139-49.

[86]   Jiang F, Bao J, Li P, Nicosia SV, Bai W: Induction of ovarian cancer cell apoptosis by 1,25-dihydroxyvitamin D3 through the down-regulation of telomerase. J Biol Chem 2004; 279(51): 53213-21.

[87]   Mantell DJ, Owens PE, Bundred NJ, Mawer EB, Canfield AE: 1 alpha,25-dihydroxyvitamin D(3) inhibits angiogenesis *in vitro* and *in vivo*. Circ Res 2000; 87(3): 214-20.

[88]   Iseki K, Tatsuta M, Uehara H, *et al.*: Inhibition of angiogenesis as a mechanism for inhibition by 1alpha-hydroxyvitamin D3 and 1,25-dihydroxyvitamin D3 of colon carcinogenesis induced by azoxymethane in Wistar rats. Int J Cancer 1999; 81(5): 730-3.

[89]   Hoyer-Hansen M, Bastholm L, Mathiasen IS, Elling F, Jaattela M: Vitamin D analog EB1089 triggers dramatic lysosomal changes and Beclin 1-mediated autophagic cell death. Cell Death Differ 2005; 12(10): 1297-309.

[90]   DeMasters GA, Gupta MS, Jones KR, *et al.*: Potentiation of cell killing by fractionated radiation and suppression of proliferative recovery in MCF-7 breast tumor cells by the Vitamin D3 analog EB 1089. J Steroid Biochem Mol Biol 2004; 92(5): 365-74.

[91]   O'Kelly J, Uskokovic M, Lemp N, Vadgama J, Koeffler HP: Novel Gemini-vitamin D3 analog inhibits tumor cell growth and modulates the Akt/mTOR signaling pathway. J Steroid Biochem Mol Biol 2006; 100(4-5): 107-16.

[92]   Krishnan AV, Srinivas S, Feldman D: Inhibition of prostaglandin synthesis and actions contributes to the beneficial effects of calcitriol in prostate cancer. Dermatoendocrinol 2009; 1(1): 7-11.

[93]   Fichera A, Little N, Dougherty U, *et al.*: A vitamin D analogue inhibits colonic carcinogenesis in the AOM/DSS model. J Surg Res 2007; 142(2): 239-45.

[94]   Aparna R, Subhashini J, Roy KR, *et al.*: Selective inhibition of cyclooxygenase-2 (COX-2) by 1alpha,25-dihydroxy-16-ene-23-yne-vitamin D3, a less calcemic vitamin D analog. Journal of Cellular Biochemistry 2008; 104(5): 1832-42.

[95]   Honma Y, Hozumi M, Abe E, *et al.*: 1 alpha,25-Dihydroxyvitamin D3 and 1 alpha-hydroxyvitamin D3 prolong survival time of mice inoculated with myeloid leukemia cells. Proceedings of the National Academy of Sciences of the United States of America 1983; 80(1): 201-4.

[96]   Zhou JY, Norman AW, Chen DL, Sun GW, Uskokovic M, Koeffler HP: 1,25-Dihydroxy-16-ene-23-yne-vitamin D3 prolongs survival time of leukemic mice. Proc Natl Acad Sci U S A 1990; 87(10): 3929-32.

[97]   Sharabani H, Izumchenko E, Wang Q, *et al.*: Cooperative antitumor effects of vitamin D3 derivatives and rosemary preparations in a mouse model of myeloid leukemia. Int J Cancer 2006; 118(12): 3012-21.

[98]   Koeffler HP, Hirji K, Itri L: 1,25-Dihydroxyvitamin D3: *in vivo* and *in vitro* effects on human preleukemic and leukemic cells. Cancer Treat Rep 1985; 69(12): 1399-407.

[99]   Richard C, Mazo E, Cuadrado MA, *et al.*: Treatment of myelodysplastic syndrome with 1.25-dihydroxy-vitamin D3. Am J Hematol 1986; 23(2): 175-8.

[100]   Metha AB, Kumaran TO, Marsh GW: Treatment of myelodysplastic syndrome with alfacalcidol. Lancet 1984; 2: 761.

[101]   Motomura S, Kanamori H, Maruta A, Kodama F, Ohkubo T: The effect of 1-hydroxyvitamin D3 for prolongation of leukemic transformation-free survival in myelodysplastic syndromes. American Journal of Hematology 1991; 38(1): 67-8.

[102]   Koeffler HP, Aslanian N, O'Kelly J: Vitamin D(2) analog (Paricalcitol; Zemplar) for treatment of myelodysplastic syndrome. Leuk Res 2005; 29(11): 1259-62.

[103]   Eisman JA, Barkla DH, Tutton PJ: Suppression of *in vivo* growth of human cancer solid tumor xenografts by 1,25-dihydroxyvitamin D3. Cancer Research 1987; 47(1): 21-5.

[104]   Tanaka Y, Wu AY, Ikekawa N, Iseki K, Kawai M, Kobayashi Y: Inhibition of HT-29 human colon cancer growth under the renal capsule of severe combined immunodeficient mice by an analogue of 1,25-dihydroxyvitamin D3, DD-003. Cancer Research 1994; 54(19): 5148-53.

[105] Akhter J, Chen X, Bowrey P, Bolton EJ, Morris DL: Vitamin D3 analog, EB1089, inhibits growth of subcutaneous xenografts of the human colon cancer cell line, LoVo, in a nude mouse model. Diseases of the Colon & Rectum 1997; 40(3): 317-21.

[106] Kumagai T, O'Kelly J, Said JW, Koeffler HP: Vitamin D2 analog 19-nor-1,25-dihydroxyvitamin D2: antitumor activity against leukemia, myeloma, and colon cancer cells. J Natl Cancer Inst 2003; 95(12): 896-905.

[107] Spina CS, Ton L, Yao M, *et al.*: Selective vitamin D receptor modulators and their effects on colorectal tumor growth. J Steroid Biochem Mol Biol 2007; 103(3-5): 757-62.

[108] Wali RK, Bissonnette M, Khare S, Hart J, Sitrin MD, Brasitus TA: 1 alpha,25-Dihydroxy-16-ene-23-yne-26,27-hexafluorocholecalciferol, a noncalcemic analogue of 1 alpha,25-dihydroxyvitamin D3, inhibits azoxymethane-induced colonic tumorigenesis. Cancer Research 1995; 55(14): 3050-4.

[109] Murillo G, Matusiak D, Benya RV, Mehta RG: Chemopreventive efficacy of 25-hydroxyvitamin D3 in colon cancer. J Steroid Biochem Mol Biol 2007; 103(3-5): 763-7.

[110] Otoshi T, Iwata H, Kitano M, *et al.*: Inhibition of intestinal tumor development in rat multi-organ carcinogenesis and aberrant crypt foci in rat colon carcinogenesis by 22-oxa-calcitriol, a synthetic analogue of 1 alpha, 25-dihydroxyvitamin D3. Carcinogenesis 1995; 16(9): 2091-7.

[111] Abe J, Nakano T, Nishii Y, Matsumoto T, Ogata E, Ikeda K: A novel vitamin D3 analog, 22-oxa-1,25-dihydroxyvitamin D3, inhibits the growth of human breast cancer *in vitro* and *in vivo* without causing hypercalcemia. Endocrinology 1991; 129(2): 832-7.

[112] Abe-Hashimoto J, Kikuchi T, Matsumoto T, Nishii Y, Ogata E, Ikeda K: Antitumor effect of 22-oxa-calcitriol, a noncalcemic analogue of calcitriol, in athymic mice implanted with human breast carcinoma and its synergism with tamoxifen. Cancer Research 1993; 53(11): 2534-7.

[113] Oikawa T, Yoshida Y, Shimamura M, Ashino-Fuse H, Iwaguchi T, Tominaga T: Antitumor effect of 22-oxa-1 alpha,25-dihydroxyvitamin D3, a potent angiogenesis inhibitor, on rat mammary tumors induced by 7,12-dimethylbenz[a]anthracene. Anti-Cancer Drugs 1991; 2(5): 475-80.

[114] Colston KW, Chander SK, Mackay AG, Coombes RC: Effects of synthetic vitamin D analogues on breast cancer cell proliferation *in vivo* and *in vitro*. Biochemical Pharmacology 1992; 44(4): 693-702.

[115] Colston KW, Mackay AG, James SY, Binderup L, Chander S, Coombes RC: EB1089: a new vitamin D analogue that inhibits the growth of breast cancer cells *in vivo* and *in vitro*. Biochemical Pharmacology 1992; 44(12): 2273-80.

[116] Murillo G, Mehta RG: Chemoprevention of chemically-induced mammary and colon carcinogenesis by 1alpha-hydroxyvitamin D5. J Steroid Biochem Mol Biol 2005; 97(1-2): 129-36.

[117] Anzano MA, Smith JM, Uskokovic MR, *et al.*: 1 alpha,25-Dihydroxy-16-ene-23-yne-26,27-hexafluorocholecalciferol (Ro24-5531), a new deltanoid (vitamin D analogue) for prevention of breast cancer in the rat. Cancer Research 1994; 54(7): 1653-6.

[118] van Weelden K, Flanagan L, Binderup L, Tenniswood M, Welsh J: Apoptotic regression of MCF-7 xenografts in nude mice treated with the vitamin D analog, EB1089. Endocrinology 1998; 139: 2103-2110.

[119] Koshizuka K, Koike M, Asou H, *et al.*: Combined effect of vitamin D3 analogs and paclitaxel on the growth of MCF-7 breast cancer cells *in vivo*. Breast Cancer Research & Treatment 1999; 53(2): 113-20.

[120] Wietrzyk J, Pelczynska M, Madej J, *et al.*: Toxicity and antineoplastic effect of (24R)-1,24-dihydroxyvitamin D3 (PRI-2191). Steroids 2004; 69(10): 629-35.

[121] Bower M, Colston KW, Stein RC, *et al.*: Topical calcipotriol treatment in advanced breast cancer [published erratum appears in Lancet 1991 Jun 29;337(8757):1618] [see comments]. Lancet 1991; 337(8743): 701-2.

[122] Gross C, Stamey T, Hancock S, Feldman D: Treatment of early recurrent prostate cancer with 1,25-dihydroxyvitamin D3 (calcitriol). J Urol 1998; 159(6): 2035-9; discussion 2039-40.

[123] Krishnan AV, Moreno J, Nonn L, Swami S, Peehl DM, Feldman D: Calcitriol as a chemopreventive and therapeutic agent in prostate cancer: role of anti-inflammatory activity. J Bone Miner Res 2007; 22 Suppl 2: V74-80.

[124] Crescioli C, Ferruzzi P, Caporali A, *et al.*: Inhibition of prostate cell growth by BXL-628, a calcitriol analogue selected for a phase II clinical trial in patients with benign prostate hyperplasia. Eur J Endocrinol 2004; 150(4): 591-603.

[125] Gross M, Kost SB, Ennis B, Stumpf W, Kumar R: Effect of 1,25-dihydroxyvitamin D3 on mouse mammary tumor (GR) cells: evidence for receptors, cellular uptake, inhibition of growth and alteration in morphology at physiologic concentrations of hormone. Journal of Bone & Mineral Research 1986; 1(5): 457-67.

[126] Schwartz GG, Hill CC, Oeler TA, Becich MJ, Bahnson RR: 1,25-Dihydroxy-16-ene-23-yne-vitamin D3 and prostate cancer cell proliferation *in vivo*. Urology 1995; 46(3): 365-9.

[127] Lucia MS, Anzano MA, Slayter MV, *et al.*: Chemopreventive activity of tamoxifen, N-(4-hydroxyphenyl)retinamide, and the vitamin D analogue RO24-5531 for adrogen-promoted carcinomas of the rat seminal vesicle and prostate. Cancer Research 1995; 55: 5621-7.

[128] Colston KW, James SY, Ofori-Kuragu EA, Binderup L, Grant AG: Vitamin D receptors and anti-proliferative effects of vitamin D derivatives in human pancreatic carcinoma cells *in vivo* and *in vitro*. British Journal of Cancer 1997; 76(8): 1017-20.

[129] Adorini L, Penna G, Amuchastegui S, *et al.*: Inhibition of prostate growth and inflammation by the vitamin D receptor agonist BXL-628 (elocalcitol). Journal of Steroid Biochemistry and Molecular Biology 2007; 103(3-5): 689-93.

[130] Osborn JL, Schwartz GG, Smith DC, Bahnson R, Day R, Trump DL: Phase II trial of oral 1,25-dihydroxyvitamin D (calcitriol) in hormone refractory prostate cancer. Urol Oncol 1995; 1(5): 195-8.

[131] Beer TM, Ryan CW, Venner PM, *et al.*: Double-blinded randomized study of high-dose calcitriol plus docetaxel compared with placebo plus docetaxel in androgen-independent prostate cancer: a report from the ASCENT Investigators. J Clin Oncol 2007; 25(6): 669-74.

[132] Kawa S, Yoshizawa K, Tokoo M, *et al.*: Inhibitory effect of 22-oxa-1,25-dihydroxyvitamin D3 on the proliferation of pancreatic cancer cell lines. Gastroenterology 1996; 110(5): 1605-13.

[133] Schwartz GG, Eads D, Naczki C, Northrup S, Chen T, Koumenis C: 19-nor-1 alpha,25-dihydroxyvitamin D2 (paricalcitol) inhibits the proliferation of human pancreatic cancer cells *in vitro* and *in vivo*. Cancer Biol Ther 2008; 7(3): 430-6.

[134] Schwartz GG, Eads D, Rao A, *et al.*: Pancreatic cancer cells express 25-hydroxyvitamin D-1 alpha-hydroxylase and their proliferation is inhibited by the prohormone 25-hydroxyvitamin D3. Carcinogenesis 2004; 25(6): 1015-26.

[135] Dixon KM, Norman AW, Sequeira VB, *et al.*: 1alpha,25(OH)-vitamin D and a nongenomic vitamin D analogue inhibit ultraviolet radiation-induced skin carcinogenesis. Cancer Prev Res (Phila) 2011; 4(9): 1485-94.

[136] Reddy CD, Patti R, Guttapalli A, *et al.*: Anticancer effects of the novel 1alpha, 25-dihydroxyvitamin D3 hybrid analog QW1624F2-2 in human neuroblastoma. J Cell Biochem 2006; 97(1): 198-206.

[137] van Ginkel PR, Yang W, Marcet MM, *et al.*: 1 alpha-Hydroxyvitamin D2 inhibits growth of human neuroblastoma. J Neurooncol 2007; 85(3): 255-62.

[138] Albert DM, Kumar A, Strugnell SA, *et al.*: Effectiveness of vitamin D analogues in treating large tumors and during prolonged use in murine retinoblastoma models. Arch Ophthalmol 2004; 122(9): 1357-62.

[139] Zhang Q, Lazar M, Molino B, *et al.*: Reduction in interaction between cGMP and cAMP in dog ventricular myocytes with hypertrophic failure. Am J Physiol Heart Circ Physiol 2005; 289(3): H1251-7.

[140] Zhang X, Nicosia SV, Bai W: Vitamin D receptor is a novel drug target for ovarian cancer treatment. Curr Cancer Drug Targets 2006; 6(3): 229-44.

[141] Nakagawa K, Sasaki Y, Kato S, Kubodera N, Okano T: 22-Oxa-1alpha,25-dihydroxyvitamin D3 inhibits metastasis and angiogenesis in lung cancer. Carcinogenesis 2005; 26(6): 1044-54.

[142] Nagpal S, Na S, Rathnachalam R: Noncalcemic actions of vitamin D receptor ligands. Endocr Rev 2005; 26(5): 662-87.

[143] Sadeghi K, Wessner B, Laggner U, *et al.*: Vitamin D3 down-regulates monocyte TLR expression and triggers hyporesponsiveness to pathogen-associated molecular patterns. Eur J Immunol 2006; 36(2): 361-70.

[144] Adorini L: Intervention in autoimmunity: the potential of vitamin D receptor agonists. Cell Immunol 2005; 233(2): 115-24.

[145] van Etten E, Mathieu C: Immunoregulation by 1,25-dihydroxyvitamin D3: basic concepts. J Steroid Biochem Mol Biol 2005; 97(1-2): 93-101.

[146] Adams JS, Hewison M: Unexpected actions of vitamin D: new perspectives on the regulation of innate and adaptive immunity. Nat Clin Pract Endocrinol Metab 2008; 4(2): 80-90.

[147] Mathieu C, Waer M, Casteels K, Laureys J, Bouillon R: Prevention of type I diabetes in NOD mice by nonhypercalcemic doses of a new structural analog of 1,25-dihydroxyvitamin D3, KH1060. Endocrinology 1995; 136(3): 866-72.

[148] Gregori S, Giarratana N, Smiroldo S, Uskokovic M, Adorini L: A 1alpha,25-dihydroxyvitamin D(3) analog enhances regulatory T-cells and arrests autoimmune diabetes in NOD mice. Diabetes 2002; 51(5): 1367-74.

[149] Van Etten E, Decallonne B, Verlinden L, Verstuyf A, Bouillon R, Mathieu C: Analogs of 1alpha,25-dihydroxyvitamin D3 as pluripotent immunomodulators. J Cell Biochem 2003; 88(2): 223-6.

[150] Lemire JM, Archer DC: 1,25-dihydroxyvitamin D3 prevents the *in vivo* induction of murine experimental autoimmune encephalomyelitis. Journal of Clinical Investigation 1991; 87(3): 1103-7.

[151]   Cantorna MT, Hayes CE, DeLuca HF: 1,25-Dihydroxyvitamin D3 reversibly blocks the progression of relapsing encephalomyelitis, a model of multiple sclerosis. Proceedings of the National Academy of Sciences of the United States of America 1996; 93(15): 7861-4.

[152]   Mattner F, Smiroldo S, Galbiati F, *et al.*: Inhibition of Th1 development and treatment of chronic-relapsing experimental allergic encephalomyelitis by a non-hypercalcemic analogue of 1,25-dihydroxyvitamin D(3). Eur J Immunol 2000; 30(2): 498-508.

[153]   van Etten E, Gysemans C, Branisteanu DD, *et al.*: Novel insights in the immune function of the vitamin D system: synergism with interferon-beta. J Steroid Biochem Mol Biol 2007; 103(3-5): 546-51.

[154]   Larsson P, Mattsson L, Klareskog L, Johnsson C: A vitamin D analogue (MC 1288) has immunomodulatory properties and suppresses collagen-induced arthritis (CIA) without causing hypercalcaemia. Clinical & Experimental Immunology 1998; 114(2): 277-83.

[155]   Cantorna MT, Hayes CE, DeLuca HF: 1,25-Dihydroxycholecalciferol inhibits the progression of arthritis in murine models of human arthritis. Journal of Nutrition 1998; 128(1): 68-72.

[156]   Lemire JM, Ince A, Takashima M: 1,25-Dihydroxyvitamin D3 attenuates the expression of experimental murine lupus of MRL/l mice. Autoimmunity 1992; 12(2): 143-8.

[157]   Koizumi T, Nakao Y, Matsui T, *et al.*: Effects of corticosteroid and 1,24R-dihydroxy-vitamin D3 administration on lymphoproliferation and autoimmune disease in MRL/MP-lpr/lpr mice. International Archives of Allergy & Applied Immunology 1985; 77(4): 396-404.

[158]   Abe J, Nakamura K, Takita Y, Nakano T, Irie H, Nishii Y: Prevention of immunological disorders in MRL/l mice by a new synthetic analogue of vitamin D3: 22-oxa-1 alpha,25-dihydroxyvitamin D3. Journal of Nutritional Science & Vitaminology 1990; 36(1): 21-31.

[159]   Cantorna MT, Munsick C, Bemiss C, Mahon BD: 1,25-Dihydroxycholecalciferol prevents and ameliorates symptoms of experimental murine inflammatory bowel disease. J Nutr 2000; 130(11): 2648-52.

[160]   Veyron P, Pamphile R, Binderup L, Touraine JL: Two novel vitamin D analogues, KH 1060 and CB 966, prolong skin allograft survival in mice. Transplant Immunology 1993; 1(1): 72-6.

[161]   Johnsson C, Binderup L, Tufveson G: The effects of combined treatment with the novel vitamin D analogue MC 1288 and cyclosporine A on cardiac allograft survival. Transplant Immunology 1995; 3(3): 245-50.

[162]   Aloia JF, Vaswani A, Yeh JK, Ellis K, Yasumura S, Cohn SH: Calcitriol in the treatment of postmenopausal osteoporosis. Am J Med 1988; 84(3 Pt 1): 401-8.

[163]   Gallagher JC, Jerpbak CM, Jee WS, Johnson KA, DeLuca HF, Riggs BL: 1,25-Dihydroxyvitamin D3: short- and long-term effects on bone and calcium metabolism in patients with postmenopausal osteoporosis. Proceedings of the National Academy of Sciences of the United States of America 1982; 79(10): 3325-9.

[164]   Ott SM, Chesnut CH, 3rd: Calcitriol treatment is not effective in postmenopausal osteoporosis. Ann Intern Med 1989; 110(4): 267-74.

[165]   Tilyard MW, Spears GF, Thomson J, Dovey S: Treatment of postmenopausal osteoporosis with calcitriol or calcium [see comments]. New England Journal of Medicine 1992; 326(6): 357-62.

[166]   Caniggia A, Nuti R, Martini G, *et al.*: Efficacy and Safety of Long-Term, Open-Label Treatment With Calcitriol in Postmenopausal Osteoporosis - a Retrospective Analysis. Current Therapeutic Research, Clinical & Experimental 1996; 57(11): 857-868.

[167]   Orimo H, Shiraki M, Hayashi T, Nakamura T: Reduced occurrence of vertebral crush fractures in senile osteoporosis treated with 1 alpha (OH)-vitamin D3. Bone Miner 1987; 3(1): 47-52.

[168]   Fujita T: Studies of osteoporosis in Japan. Metabolism 1990; 39(4 Suppl 1): 39-42.

[169]   Ringe JD, Farahmand P, Schacht E, Rozehnal A: Superiority of a combined treatment of Alendronate and Alfacalcidol compared to the combination of Alendronate and plain vitamin D or Alfacalcidol alone in established postmenopausal or male osteoporosis (AAC-Trial). Rheumatol Int 2007; 27(5): 425-34.

[170]   Tsurukami H, Nakamura T, Suzuki K, Sato K, Higuchi Y, Nishii Y: A novel synthetic vitamin D analogue, 2 beta-(3-hydroxypropoxy)1 alpha, 25-dihydroxyvitamin D3 (ED-71), increases bone mass by stimulating the bone formation in normal and ovariectomized rats. Calcified Tissue International 1994; 54(2): 142-9.

[171]   Tanaka Y, Nakamura T, Nishida S, *et al.*: Effects of a synthetic vitamin D analog, ED-71, on bone dynamics and strength in cancellous and cortical bone in prednisolone-treated rats. Journal of Bone & Mineral Research 1996; 11(3): 325-36.

[172]   Matsumoto T, Kubodera N: ED-71, a new active vitamin D3, increases bone mineral density regardless of serum 25(OH)D levels in osteoporotic subjects. Journal of Steroid Biochemistry and Molecular Biology 2007; 103(3-5): 584-6.

[173] Shevde NK, Plum LA, Clagett-Dame M, Yamamoto H, Pike JW, DeLuca HF: A potent analog of 1a,25-dihydroxyvitamin D3 selectively induced bone formation. Proceedings of the National Academy of Sciences of the United States of America 2002; 99: 13487-91.

[174] Plum LA, Fitzpatrick LA, Ma X, *et al.*: 2MD, a new anabolic agent for osteoporosis treatment. Osteoporos Int 2006; 17(5): 704-15.

[175] Ke HZ, Qi H, Crawford DT, *et al.*: A new vitamin D analog, 2MD, restores trabecular and cortical bone mass and strength in ovariectomized rats with established osteopenia. J Bone Miner Res 2005; 20(10): 1742-55.

[176] Brown AJ, Slatopolsky E: Vitamin D analogs: therapeutic applications and mechanisms for selectivity. Molecular Aspects of Medicine 2008; 29(6): 433-52.

CHAPTER 7

Future Perspectives

J. Ruth Wu-Wong[*]

Department of Pharmacy Practice, University of Illinois, USA

Abstract: Emerging evidence suggests that vitamin D plays important roles in modulating cardiovascular, immunological, metabolic and other functions. However, numerous questions remain unanswered about the vitamin D-VDR axis. For example, is vitamin D a vitamin? Is it a hormone? Or is it both vitamin and hormone depending on whether it is the precursor or the active metabolite? Current clinical practices focus on measuring 25(OH)D deficiency in the blood. One important question that needs to be addressed is whether 25(OH)D is a proper marker for gauging VDR activation or not. It is well recognized that 25(OH)D is a precursor of the active form of vitamin D, calcitriol; 25(OH)D itself is not effective in activating VDR. In addition, studies have shown that, beside deficiency in vitamin D or 25(OH)D, many other factors such as disease, aging, gene polymorphism, *etc.* also impact vitamin D metabolism and VDR activation. Is there a need to develop biomarkers that can measure the deficiency in VDR activation at the molecular level so that the root of the problem can be properly corrected? Although vitamin D and its analogs are potentially useful for preventing and treating various diseases, their usage at this point is still rather limited. It is partially due to the fact that there is no way to distinguish whether the lack of effect of vitamin D and its analogs in clinical studies is due to inadequate activation of VDR or a general lack of efficacy. Biomarkers and assays to determine deficiency in VDR activation will be very useful. Another potential issue is that current on-the-market vitamin D analogs used to treat diseases such as hyperparathyroidism secondary to chronic kidney disease, psoriasis and osteoporosis have narrow therapeutic index and considerable side effects. New vitamin D analogs that have a wider therapeutic index without the hypercalcemic liability will allow the expanded usage of this class of drugs into new indications. As the field continues to evolve and new technology advances, the potential of vitamin D and its analogs for the prevention and treatment of various disorders will likely be realized in the near future.

Keywords: Aging, biomarker, disease prevention, hormone, liver, kidney, new VDR agonists, novel analogs, side effect, therapeutic index, VDR activation, VDR polymorphism, vitamin D dose.

INTRODUCTION

News about the diverse effects of vitamin D seems to show up everywhere during the past few years. A series of articles appeared in *USA Today* in the first six months of 2008 talking about the link between low blood levels of vitamin D and increased risk for various diseases such as cancers, autoimmune diseases, cardiovascular problems and particularly heart-related deaths. Then there was a CNN report on Vitamin D in 2009. In the 2010 January issue of "Better Homes and Gardens", there was a mentioning that "recent research has found that a deficiency of vitamin D, the so-called sunshine vitamin, may increase risk of osteoporosis, breast cancer, hypertension and multiple sclerosis". As discussed in previous chapters, numerous other reports also linked vitamin D deficiency to various health issues including skeletal disorders, valvular calcification [1], chronic kidney disease [2], metabolic disturbances in polycystic ovary syndrome [3], fatal cancer [4], immune disorders such as multiple sclerosis [5], *etc.*

Clearly the public is becoming more aware of the benefits of vitamin D beyond its traditional role in bone health. In 2010, the official vitamin D recommendations were updated for the first time since 1997. As eloquently described by other authors in this eBook, vitamin D receptor, one of the steroid nuclear receptor superfamily, is present in more than 30 tissues in the human body and likely involved in modulating many different functions beyond regulation of mineral homeostasis.

*Address correspondence to J. Ruth Wu-Wong: Department of Pharmacy Practice, University of Illinois, Chicago, IL. 60612, USA; E-mail: jrwuwong@uic.edu

However, although the vitamin D field has been around for several decades, many questions remain unanswered, and more work will be needed in the future in order to reap the full benefit of vitamin D and its analogs. In this chapter, several of these questions and potential approaches to answer them will be discussed.

THE TERMINOLOGY: IS VITAMIN D A VITAMIN?

Although this issue has been discussed in previous chapters, it is worthy of another mentioning here. According to Webster's online dictionary, a vitamin is "an organic compound that cannot be synthesized (at all, or in quantities that meet all needs) by a given organism and must be taken (in trace quantities) with food for that organism's continued good health". By this definition, vitamin D shall not belong to the "vitamin" category since we humans can make vitamin D_3 in the skin by simply exposing to sunshine, which will meet all of our vitamin D need under normal circumstances.

Besides making vitamin D_3 in the skin by exposing to sunshine, humans can also acquire vitamin D_2 or D_3 *via* food or vitamin D supplement. However, vitamin D_3 is not immediately active, but needs to be converted to 25-hydroxyvitamin D_3 ($25(OH)D_3$) by 25-hydroxylase in the liver, followed by further hydroxylation by 25-hydroxyvitamin D_3 1-alpha-hydroxylase (CYP27B1, 1α-hydroxylase) to form the active hormone, $1\alpha,25$-dihydroxyvitamin D_3 ($1\alpha,25(OH)_2D_3$ or calcitriol). The second hydroxylation step by CYP27B1 occurs mainly in the kidney, which results in the production of circulating (endocrine) calcitriol. Extra-renal calcitriol synthesis can also occur in other cells and tissues but it does not significantly contribute to endocrine calcitriol levels and is considered primarily to have an autocrine and/or paracrine function [6, 7]. The binding of calcitriol ($1\alpha,25(OH)_2D_3$) or its analogs to the vitamin D receptor (VDR), a nuclear receptor, activates VDR to recruit cofactors to form a complex that binds to vitamin D response elements in the promoter region of target genes to regulate gene transcription [6, 8]. Please refer to previous chapters for more detailed descriptions regarding the synthesis of vitamin D and the VDR signaling pathway.

It is now well recognized by researchers in the field that the active form of vitamin D is actually a hormone that activates a nuclear receptor, just like estrogen and androgen that activate their target nuclear receptors. However, to promote the idea that vitamin D is not a vitamin often evokes criticism and objection. After all, even the NIH "Office of Dietary Supplements" website (http://dietary-supplements.info.nih.gov/factsheets/vitamind.asp#h3. Accessed April 2, 2011) stated that "the Vitamin D is a fat-soluble vitamin that is naturally present in very few foods, added to others, and available as a dietary supplement", although the website did mention that vitamin D is also produced endogenously when ultraviolet rays from sunlight strike the skin and trigger vitamin D synthesis.

Since the terminology "vitamin D" has been around for so long and is so well received, it is probably not possible to try to change it at this point. The alternative perhaps is to continue to provide information about the true nature of the vitamin D system including its hormone characteristics and widespread functions. It is one of the reasons why this eBook was conceived. We sincerely hope that this eBook will help educating students, researchers and/or the general public about the importance of the "vitamin D hormone".

VITAMIN D DEFICIENCY: HOW MUCH VITAMIN D IS NEEDED TO MAINTAIN GOOD HEALTH?

As discussed in the previous chapters, recent clinical observations have generated substantial excitements in the health care community and also among the general public regarding the use of vitamin D and its analogs to prevent and/or treat various diseases. One key question that remains unanswered is: what is the optimal dose of vitamin D?

According to the NIH "Office of Dietary Supplements" website, most people meet their vitamin D needs through exposure to sunlight. However, season, geographic latitude, time of day, cloud cover, smog, skin melanin content, and sunscreen can affect UVB radiation exposure and vitamin D synthesis (http://dietary-supplements.info.nih.gov/factsheets/vitamind.asp#h3. Accessed April 2, 2011). Therefore, vitamin D supplementation in addition to sun exposure is often necessary. In 2010 the U.S. Institute of Medicine

(IOM) updated their recommendations on the dietary reference intake of vitamin D for the different life stage groups with minimal sun exposure (see Chapter 4 for more details).

However many experts believe that even 600-800 IU/day is inadequate and 2000 IU/day shall be the dose for the general public. Yet, no solid data exist to support either recommendation. One major issue associated with the difficulty in determining the optimal daily dose of vitamin D supplementation has to do with the lack of tools and/or technologies available in the vitamin D field.

Intuitively one would think that the serum $1,25(OH)_2D$ level is a good indicator for the vitamin D status since $1,25(OH)_2D$ (calcitriol, $1,25(OH)_2D_3$) is the active form of vitamin D that is responsible for activating the receptor and initiating the VDR signaling pathway. However, the circulating calcitriol level has never been considered a good indicator of vitamin D status for a variety of reasons. First, $1,25(OH)_2D$ has a relatively short half-life *vs.* $25(OH)D$. Secondly, the determination of calcitriol in the blood is quite challenging due to its low level. In healthy individuals, the average level of $25(OH)D$ in blood circulation is ~30 ng/mL (~75 nM), while the level of calcitriol is maintained at 1 - 45 pg/ml (equivalent to 0.002 - 0.1 nM). Thirdly, there is a lack of correlation between the serum $1,25(OH)_2D$ level and the vitamin D status. Unless the vitamin D deficiency is extremely severe, a decrease in the serum $1,25(OH)_2D$ level is usually not seen. In healthy individuals, vitamin D deficiency results in a compensatory increase in parathyroid hormone (PTH), which increases the renal production of calcitriol. Consequently, serum calcitriol levels are often normal or even elevated in people with vitamin D deficiency. Fourthly, although the VDR signaling pathway is dependent on the availability of calcitriol, it is not known whether there is a correlation between the serum calcitriol level and the calcitriol concentration at the cellular and/or tissue sites. It is also not well established what the optimal blood $1,25(OH)_2D$ level shall be in order to activate VDR to maintain good health.

The serum calcitriol concentration is tightly regulated. In addition to parathyroid hormone, calcium, and phosphate, a host of proteins and enzymes such as vitamin D-binding protein (DBP), the putative liver 25-hydroxylase (CYP27A1), CYP27B1 and CYP24A1 (1,25-dihydroxyvitamin D_3 24-hydroxylase or 24-hydroxylase), along with others such as megalin (an endocytic receptor responsible for the resorption of DBP in the kidney) and FGF-23 (known to inhibit CYP27B1), all play a role in maintaining a balance among the vitamin D, $25(OH)D$ and $1,25(OH)_2D$ levels in blood circulation. However, since CYP27B1 is present at various cells and tissues, presumably cells and tissues have the ability to make calcitriol locally and the calcitriol concentration in cells and tissues, at least in theory, can be much higher than the blood calcitriol level.

Therefore, for many years up to the present moment, serum concentration of $25(OH)D$ is considered a better indicator of vitamin D status. The serum $25(OH)D$ has a fairly long circulating half-life of 15 days, and is relatively easier to measure. It seems to correlate well with the vitamin D produced cutaneously and obtained from food and supplements [9, 10].

However, several issues exist when using the serum $25(OH)D$ levels as an indicator for vitamin D metabolism. First, the serum $25(OH)D$ levels do not indicate the amount of vitamin D stored in other body tissues. Secondly, even though it is easier to determine the serum $25(OH)D$ than the $1,25(OH)_2D$ levels, considerable variability exists among the various assays used by different laboratories. A standard reference material for $25(OH)D$ that became available in July 2009 shall now permit standardization of values across laboratories (National Institute of Standards and Technology. NIST releases vitamin D standard reference material, 2009). Thirdly and perhaps the most difficult issue to address is: how do we know the serum $25(OH)D$ levels accurately reflect VDR activation and its signaling pathways at the molecular level?

Many consider a level of $25(OH)D$ at ≤15 ng/mL indicating vitamin D deficiency, while a level between 15 – 30 ng/mL is borderline and a level more than 30 ng/mL is adequate. However, these $25(OH)D$ levels were arbitrarily derived from the distribution of $25(OH)D$ in the normal population. Simply put, although most studies seem to suggest that $25(OH)D$ levels at 30-40 ng/mL are "adequate for bone and overall health in healthy individuals" according to the NIH "Office of Dietary Supplements" website [11], the fact is that the optimal blood level of $25(OH)D$ is not known. Assuming a correlation between low $25(OH)D$ levels and increased risk for poor health is true, then in theory vitamin D supplementation shall raise $25(OH)D$ levels and reduce risks for various diseases. However, as pointed out in previous chapters, discrepancy exists regarding the beneficial effects of vitamin D supplementation on hypertension, diabetes, inflammation markers and mortality. Even on the very basic question of whether vitamin D supplementation raises serum 25(OH)D levels, there is inconsistency from study to study. Truly the question regarding whether the serum 25(OH)D level is a good indicator for VDR function remains to be addressed.

Perhaps we have been asking the wrong question all along. Is the deficiency in VDR activation, rather than vitamin D, 25(OH)D, and/or calcitriol deficiency, a more important etiologic factor for the increased risk for various disorders? If the answer to this question is "yes", then how can we determine deficiency in VDR activation?

Unfortunately this question has no satisfactory answers at this point. In chronic kidney disease (CKD) patients, the serum PTH level seems to indicate a problem with VDR activation since PTH is one of the direct target genes for VDR. When vitamin D and/or VDR agonists (VDRAs) are used to treat secondary hyperparathyroidism in CKD, PTH suppression is a useful endpoint to indicate whether the patient responds to therapy or not. Outside of PTH suppression, currently there is no marker available to gauge the efficacy of vitamin D and/or VDRA therapy. For example, controlled interventional trials with vitamin D supplement yielded no consistent results regarding the prevention of extravertebral fractures [12]. It is not known whether the lack of effect is due to the low level of vitamin D used in the study or a general lack of efficacy of vitamin D supplement towards the prevention of fractures.

Considering the important role of VDR in many physiological functions, vitamin D and its analogs can be one of the cheapest, most effective ways to improve the health of the general public and to reduce the health care cost. It will be of tremendous value if biomarkers can be identified and assays developed to determine deficiency in VDR activation at the molecular level. Only after that, the potential of vitamin D and its analogs for the prevention and treatment of various disorders can be fully realized.

VITAMIN D AND ITS ANALOGS FOR DISEASE PREVENTION/TREATMENT

As described in the previous chapters, numerous pre-clinical and clinical studies have suggested that vitamin D and its analogs are useful for the prevention and treatment of various diseases.

The Usage of Vitamin D and Its Analogs

It is important to note that vitamin D is usually sold as a supplement without a need for prescription except for a high dose form (50,000 IU) of cholecalciferol (vitamin D$_3$) or ergocalciferol (vitamin D$_2$), but vitamin D analogs such as calcitriol, alfacalcidol, doxercalciferol and paricalcitol are drugs that require prescriptions. The applications of vitamin D and its analogs to prevent and/or treat disease also are not the same. Table **1** is an attempt to summarize the usage of vitamin D and its analogs for the prevention and treatment of several diseases supported by scientific evidences and clinical experiences.

Table 1: Diseases treated with vitamin D and its analogs supported by scientific evidence and clinical experiences

Disease	Causes/Symptoms	Treatment
Familial hypophosphatemia	Inherited disorder: impaired phosphate transport in the blood and diminished vitamin D metabolism in the kidneys leading to low blood levels of phosphate in the blood	Calcitriol
Fanconi syndrome-related hypophosphatemia	A defect of the proximal tubules of the kidney, which is associated with renal tubular acidosis	Ergocalciferol
Hyperparathyroidism due to low vitamin D levels	Elevated serum parathyroid hormone; enlarged parathyroid gland	Vitamin D
Hyperparathyroidism secondary to chronic kidney disease	Elevated serum parathyroid hormone and enlarged parathyroid gland due to reduced kidney function in converting 25(OH)D to 1,25(OH)$_2$D	Cholecalciferol or ergocalciferol in early stage CKD; alfacalcidol, calcitriol, doxercalciferol, paricalcitol in Stage 4/5 CKD

Table 1: cont….

Hypocalcemia due to hypoparathyroidism	Hypoparathyroidism (low blood levels of parathyroid hormone) due to surgical removal of the parathyroid glands.	Calcitriol or ergocalciferol
Osteomalacia (adult rickets)	Severe vitamin D deficiency leading to loss of bone mineral content ("hypomineralization") and bone pain, muscle weakness, and osteomalacia (soft bones).	Vitamin D
Psoriasis	Abnormal skin cell growth and skin plaques due to a form of autoimmune disorder	Becocalcidiol, calcipotriene, tacalcitol
Rickets	Bone disorders in children due to vitamin D deficiency	Calcitriol (for CKD patients), cholecalciferol, ergocalciferol

In addition, there is adequate scientific evidence to support that vitamin D and its analogs are useful to prevent and/or treat viral and bacterial infection such as influenza and tuberculosis [13-15], musculoskeletal disorders [16, 17], osteoporosis, renal osteodystrophy (bone problems associated with chronic kidney disease).

Studies also suggest, although evidence is not as robust, that vitamin D and its analogs may be useful to reduce anticonvulsant-induced osteomalacia and to prevent some forms of cancer such as breast cancer and colorectal cancer [18, 19], diabetes [20, 21], high blood pressure [22], hypertriglyceridemia, immune disorders [23-25], multiple sclerosis, myelodysplastic syndrome, proximal myopathy, seasonal affective disorder, senile warts, skin pigmentation disorders (pigmented lesions).

Issues Associated With the Usage of Vitamin D and Its Analogs

Controversies do exist regarding the usefulness of vitamin D supplementation and/or vitamin D analogs to prevent and/or treat diseases. For example, Scragg *et al.* [26] gave individuals from general practitioner age-sex registers in Cambridge (UK) a single oral dose of 2.5 mg cholecalciferol, and followed them up at 5 weeks later. Neither blood pressure nor serum cholesterol concentrations were altered. However, the serum 25(OH)D levels only increased by 7.2 nmol/l to 18 nmol/l (equivalent to ~7.2 ng/mL) in that study. As a comparison, when 148 elderly women were supplemented with 1200 mg calcium plus 800 IU (20 μg) vitamin D_3 or 1200 mg calcium alone daily for 8 weeks, the group with vitamin D_3 + calcium resulted in a 72% increase in serum 25(OH)D (from 10 to 17 ng/mL), a 17% decrease in serum PTH, a 9.3% decrease in systolic blood pressure (SBP), and a 5.4% decrease in heart rate [27].

Although controlled interventional trials with vitamin D supplement (and calcium) yielded no consistent results in terms of the prevention of extravertebral fractures [12], treatment with VDRAs such as alfacalcidol seems to exert better effects [28]. This observation is further supported by a comparative meta-analysis [29], in which 14 trials were included with 21,268 patients randomized to native vitamin D, VDRAs, or placebo. When focusing on studies featuring the highest methodological quality, a statistically significant lower level of risk for falls was observed in the VDRA group *vs.* the native vitamin D group (a 3.5-fold difference). A similar observation was made by MacLean *et al.* [30] looking at bone fractures. Cancer is another example where controversies exist regarding the usefulness of vitamin D supplementation and/or vitamin D and its analogs, as pointed out in the previous chapters.

The reasons for these controversies are not apparent. As mentioned earlier, vitamin D_3 synthesized in the skin is not immediately active, but needs to be converted to $25(OH)D_3$ in the liver, followed by further hydroxylation by CYP27B1 to form the active hormone, $1\alpha,25(OH)_2D_3$ (calcitriol), which then binds to VDR to activate the VDR signaling pathway. One possible explanation for the inconsistent results may be related to the existence of polymorphisms in genes involved in the vitamin D-VDR axis.

Heist *et al.* [31] examined survival in 294 patients with advanced non-small cell lung cancer, and found that certain VDR polymorphisms showed an association with better survival. Similarly Li *et al.* [32] examined the associations between 25(OH)D levels and the risk for prostate cancer and found that the genetic polymorphism with the presence of a less functional allele of the VDR appeared to be associated with a higher risk of aggressive prostate cancer in patients with lower 25(OH)D levels. Evidence exists to show that, besides VDR, CYP27B1 polymorphism plays a role as well. Yang and Xiong [33] reported that CYP27B1 gene promoter polymorphism, especially in the -1260A/C region, is associated with increased risk for autoimmune thyroid diseases in Chinese Han population. A similar finding was previously reported by Lopez and Zwermann [34] in a German population that the allelic variation of the promoter (-1260) C/A polymorphism in CYP27B1 is associated with increased risks for endocrine autoimmune diseases such as Addison's disease, Hashimoto's thyroiditis, Graves' disease and type 1 diabetes mellitus. Beside VDR and CYP27B1, polymorphisms of other proteins involved in the vitamin D system may also impact VDR functionality. As mentioned above, a host of proteins and enzymes including DBP, CYP27B1, CYP24A1, megalin, and FGF-23 all play a role in the vitamin D system. Presumably polymorphisms may exist in any of the proteins in the VDR signaling pathway, leading to different outcomes depending on the patient populations treated with vitamin D and/or its analogs in the clinical studies.

Beside polymorphism, other factors such as aging and diseases may impact vitamin D metabolism. It has been shown that the capacity for UVB-induced cutaneous synthesis of vitamin D goes down at older age [35]. On the other hand, both hypervitaminosis D due to an increased CYP27B1 activity and a complete or partial lack of vitamin D action (VDR-/- mice and CYP27B1-/-) result in premature aging. It seems that there is an optimal concentration of vitamin D in delaying aging phenomena [36]. Lee *et al.* [37] reported that an inverse relationship exists between 25(OH)D levels and metabolic syndrome, which is independent of several confounders and PTH, and the relationship is partly explained by insulin resistance. Obesity has also been shown to be associated with vitamin D deficiency [38]. However, although interesting observations suggest that the vitamin D system is impacted by various factors, the clinical significance of these observations warrants further study.

When Liver and Kidney Are Diseased

Since the active hormonal form of vitamin D is mainly formed after the precursor is further processed in liver and kidney, it is reasonable to assume that people of reduced liver and/or kidney function may not be able to activate vitamin D properly, leading to defective function in the VDR signaling pathway.

Some studies show that there is interaction between liver and the vitamin D system. Hu *et al.* [39] reported that in female BALB/C mice administered ConA to induce acute immunological liver injury, calcitriol significantly decreased the serum alanine transaminase levels and markedly attenuated the histological liver damage. The beneficial effect of calcitriol was associated with: (i) inhibition of CD4(+) T cell activation; (ii) reduction of interferon-gamma (IFN-gamma) and elevation of both IL-4 and IL-5 in splenocytes; and (iii) elimination of activated T cells by increasing VDR mRNA and protein expression in the spleen.

In the clinical setting, Arteh *et al.* [40] reported that, in 118 consecutive patients with chronic liver disease (43 with hepatitis C cirrhosis, 57 with hepatitis C but no cirrhosis, 18 with nonhepatitis C-related cirrhosis), 25(OH)D deficiency is universal (92%), and at least one-third of them suffer from severe vitamin D deficiency (<7 ng/mL). African American females are at highest risk of vitamin D deficiency. Petta *et al.* [41] demonstrated that genotype 1 chronic hepatitis C (G1 CHC) patients had low 25(OH)D serum levels, possibly because of reduced CYP27A1 expression. Furthermore, low serum 25(OH)D level was related to severe fibrosis and low responsiveness to interferon-based therapy in G1 CHC patients. Targher *et al.* [42] reported that, in 60 consecutive patients with biopsy-proven non-alcoholic fatty liver disease (NAFLD) *vs.* 60 healthy controls of comparable age, sex and body mass index (BMI), NAFLD patients had a marked decrease in winter serum 25(OH)D concentrations, and decreased 25(OH)D concentrations were closely associated with the histological severity of hepatic steatosis, necroinflammation and fibrosis. Metabolic syndrome occurred more frequently among NAFLD patients, but it is not known whether vitamin D may play a role in the development and progression of NAFLD.

Numerous evidences demonstrate that the kidney plays a critical role in the vitamin D axis, and at the same time deficient VDR activation may be an important factor for the development and progression of chronic kidney disease (CKD).

CKD patients experience abnormal vitamin D metabolism and have abnormalities in many other parameters such as calcium, phosphorus, PTH, bone, *etc.*, which can be related to deficient VDR signaling. Levin *et al.* [43] reported from an outpatient cohort cross-sectional study conducted in 153 centers that, when kidney function declines in patients with CKD, a decrease in the serum calcitriol level is the first to occur, before other changes in serum calcium, phosphate, PTH or 25(OH)D can be observed. Significant differences in the mean and median values of calcitriol and PTH are seen across deciles of estimated glomerular filtration rate (eGFR), but the rise in PTH is only observed following a decrease in calcitriol.

It is well documented that VDR regulates PTH expression at the transcriptional level directly and also indirectly regulates PTH *via* calcium absorption. Calcitriol (the endogenous VDR activator) and its analogs such as alfacalcidol, paricalcitol and doxercalciferol have been used to treat hyperparathyroidism secondary to CKD for many years [44]; the structures of several of these drugs are shown in previous chapters. Controversies exist regarding whether vitamin D supplementation or 25(OH)D (that requires a functional kidney for activation) is as effective as active vitamin D analogs in treating late stages of CKD patients. Although vitamin D (ergocalciferol or cholecalciferol) is able to reduce PTH in early stages of CKD, native vitamin D therapy seems inadequate for late stages of CKD [45]. A study by Dusso *et al.* [46] examined the efficacy of 25(OH)D on reducing PTH in hemodialysis patients, and found that 200 μg per day of 25(OH)D given orally for two weeks increased serum 25(OH)D and $1,25(OH)_2D$ levels, but did not cause any significant change in PTH. It seems that ergocalciferol or cholecalciferol can increase 25(OH)D and/or $1,25(OH)_2D$ levels and suppress PTH in Stage 3 CKD patients, but has no significant effects in late stages (Stage 4/5) of CKD [47, 48]. Nevertheless, these results demonstrate that there is a direct correlation between renal function and vitamin D metabolism.

In preclinical studies, calcitriol was shown to reduce urinary protein and attenuate glomerular cells proliferation in anti-Thy-1.1. nephritis rats, an experimental model of mesangial proliferative glomerulonephritis [49]. In a mouse model of obstructive nephropathy characterized by predominant tubulointerstitial lesions, paricalcitol reduced infiltration of T cells and macrophages in the obstructed kidney, accompanied by a decreased expression of RANTES and TNF-alpha [50]. In the same model paricalcitol treatment resulted in a reduced interstitial volume, decreased collagen deposition, and repressed mRNA expression of fibronectin and type I and type III collagens. In the 5/6 nephrectomized uremic (NX) rat model, $1,25(OH)_2$-22-oxa-calcitriol, another active vitamin D analog, significantly suppressed urinary albumin excretion, prevented increases in serum creatinine and serum urea nitrogen, and inhibited glomerular cell number, glomerulosclerosis ratio and glomerular volume [51]. Mizobuchi *et al.* [52] reported that there was improvement in creatinine clearance and the excretion of urinary protein in NX rats treated with enalapril, paricalcitol or enalapril + paricalcitol. Interestingly, enalapril normalized blood pressure but paricalcitol had no effect. Another study by Freudlich *et al.* [53] reported that glomerular and tubulointerstitial damage, hypertension, proteinuria, and the deterioration of renal function resulting from renal ablation were significantly less in NX rats receiving paricalcitol.

In clinical studies, Agarwal *et al.* [54] showed that, in three double-blind, randomized, placebo-controlled studies to evaluate the safety and efficacy of oral paricalcitol in 220 stage 3 and 4 CKD patients with SHPT, 51% of the paricalcitol patients (*vs.* 25% placebo patients) had reduction in proteinuria. Proteinuria is a marker of cardiovascular and renal disease in patients with CKD, and reduction in proteinuria has been associated with improved cardiovascular and renal outcomes. Another paper by the same group [55] reported that, in CKD Stage 2/3 patients, paricalcitol reduced albuminuria and C-reactive protein independent of PTH or blood pressure. In an open-label prospective uncontrolled study [56], patients with immunoglobulin A (IgA) nephropathy were treated with calcitriol for 12 weeks on top of angiotensin-converting enzyme-inhibitor or angiotensin receptor blocker therapy. Calcitriol therapy resulted in a significant decrease in proteinuria with time, and also a progressive decrease in urine protein-creatinine ratio. In a recent randomized controlled trial studying pre-dialysis CKD patients, the VITAL (Selective Vitamin D Receptor Activator (Paricalcitol) for Albuminuria Lowering) trial [57], 281 patients with type 2 diabetes and albuminuria receiving ACE inhibitors or ARBs were treated for 24 weeks with placebo, 1 μg/day or 2 μg/day of paricalcitol. The primary endpoint was the percentage change in geometric mean urinary albumin-to-creatinine ratio (UACR) from baseline to last measurement for the combined paricalcitol groups *vs.* the placebo group. Change in UACR was –3% in the placebo group, –16% in the combined paricalcitol groups, –14% in the 1 μg paricalcitol group, and –20% in the 2 μg paricalcitol group. Furthermore, patients on 2 μg paricalcitol showed an early, sustained reduction in UACR, ranging from –18% to –28% (p = 0.014 *vs.* placebo). Regression analysis on log-transformed UACR showed that 84% reduction in UACR was from the direct effect of 2 μg paricalcitol and 16% was due to the indirect effect of paricalcitol on reducing systolic blood pressure. The authors concluded that adding 2 μg/day paricalcitol on top of ACE inhibitors or ARBs safely lowered residual albuminuria in patients with diabetic nephropathy, and that VDRAs could be a novel approach to lower residual renal risk in diabetic CKD.

What to Treat?

The observations that factors such as polymorphism, aging and diseases impact vitamin D metabolism raise additional questions. For example, Holick *et al.* [35] showed that the capacity for UVB-induced cutaneous synthesis of vitamin D goes down at older age. How about the effect of aging on the function of CYP27B1 and/or VDR? If the expression and/or activity of CYP27B1 or VDR also decrease as a result of aging, then taking vitamin D supplement may not be adequate, and a vitamin D analog that activates the "weakened" VDR directly may be necessary. Regarding polymorphism, it seems that the CYP27B1 enzyme in some individuals may not be functioning as effectively as that in others. If so, giving the same amount of vitamin D may not necessarily result in a similar increase in the $1,25(OH)_2D$ level. In addition, the VDR functionality may also be different. Thus, even with the same level of $1,25(OH)_2D$, the actual activation of VDR and its signaling pathway may not be the same. The impact of disease is another area of interest. As mentioned above, CYP27B1 functionality is greatly reduced in CKD. However, evidence also suggests that VDR expression and binding affinity for calcitriol may also decrease in CKD [58]. All these questions in the field require further investigations.

The understanding that many factors affect the vitamin D system makes one wonder whether activating VDR adequately shall be the goal for treatment rather than correcting vitamin D, 25(OH)D or $1,25(OH)_2D$ deficiency. However, it brings us back to the question mentioned earlier: What markers are indicative of whether VDR is adequately activated? In CKD with secondary hyperparathyroidism, PTH suppression is a useful endpoint to indicate whether the patient responds to vitamin D analog therapy or not. Outside of PTH suppression, currently there is no marker available to gauge the efficacy of vitamin D and/or VDRA therapy. In order to answer many of the questions about how polymorphism, aging and/or other factors affect vitamin D metabolism, indeed there is a need to develop new tools/methods to help gauge VDR functionality.

DIFFERENT FORMS OF VITAMIN D AND ITS ANALOGS

Vitamin D currently sold as a supplement without a need for prescription is available in two distinct forms, vitamin D_2 and vitamin D_3. Both are referred to as vitamin D although they are different in their origins and metabolism. Vitamin D_3 is the one produced in the human skin with sunlight exposure, while Vitamin D_2 is usually derived from plants. The two forms are generally regarded as equivalent and interchangeable likely due to the fact that, in the early years of research, bioassays were used to establish the amount of vitamin D required for recalcification of the epiphyseal end of tibiae in rats. However, as pointed out in previous chapters, more recent studies demonstrate that vitamins D_2 and D_3 are not the same in humans. For example, Armas *et al.* [59] compared the two forms of vitamin D in 20 healthy male volunteers over a period of 28 days and found that, by measuring the area under the curve of the rise in 25(OH)D above baseline, vitamins D_2 potency is less than one third that of vitamins D_3. In addition, other studies have shown that vitamins D_2 is metabolized to various substances in the body, some of which are not normally present in humans, although these metabolites have not been shown to be toxic [60]. Some experts in the field have even suggested that vitamins D_2 should not be used as a nutrient suitable for supplementation or fortification.

Regarding the active form of vitamin D, calcitriol and its analogs, these drugs have been tested extensively in numerous preclinical animal models and used clinically for >20 years to treat various diseases including hyperparathyroidism secondary to CKD. Results from both preclinical and clinical studies seem to suggest that these different VDR agonists (VDRAs), although structurally rather similar, behave quite differently.

For example, paricalcitol has been shown in the 5/6 nephrectomized uremic rats and also in CKD patients to have a 3-4x wider therapeutic index (by comparing PTH suppressing efficacy *vs.* hypercalcemic toxicity) than calcitriol [61, 62]. Vascular calcification is another area where different VDRAs may have different effects, although existing data were mainly from preclinical studies. Hirata *et al.* [51] showed that calcitriol induced vascular calcification in the NX uremic rats, while $1,25(OH)_2$-22-oxa-calcitriol (OCT), an analog of calcitriol, did not show any effect. They also showed that OCT at a high dose (6.25 µg/kg) raised serum Ca^{2+}, Pi and CaxPi levels to the same level as calcitriol at 0.125 µg/kg, but only calcitriol induced aortic calcification. Others [63-68] found that calcitriol, paricalcitol and doxercalciferol exhibited different effects on vascular calcification in the NX uremic rat model that calcitriol and doxercalciferol increased the aortic Ca^{2+} content more than paricalcitol.

One of the most important, yet controversial, findings during the past few years is about the survival benefits of VDRAs for CKD patients. Table **2** is a summary of human studies examining mortality and VDRA therapy in CKD patients. The common theme from these studies is that VDRAs, although mainly prescribed to treat SHPT, were associated with a significant survival benefit for CKD patients, either on dialysis or pre-dialysis. Also, the survival benefit for CKD patients seems to be independent of mineral metabolism and PTH. An interesting observation is that the survival benefit may be different for different VDRAs with paricalcitol associated with better survival than calcitriol [69]. One major issue of the studies listed in Table **2** is that all of them are observational studies.

The potential "differential" effect of VDRAs is a topic of interest and importance, but at the same time continues to be a source for controversies and debates. For example, what is the mechanism of action for the differential effects of different VDRAs on vascular calcification or on raising serum calcium? Some studies have attempted to answer these questions. Mizobuchi *et al.* [67] showed that calcitriol or doxercalciferol treatment increased the mRNA and protein expression of the bone-related markers Runx2 and osteocalcin in the aorta whereas paricalcitol did not, which may explain why paricalcitol has lesser effects on vascular calcification. Nakane *et al.* [70] reported from *ex vivo* and *in vitro* studies that paricalcitol has lesser effects than calcitriol or doxercalciferol (and its active form, $1,25(OH)_2D_2$) on inducing the expression of genes encoding calbindin 3 and TRPV6 (transient receptor potential cation channel subfamily V member 6), and on stimulating intestinal active calcium transport, which may explain why paricalcitol is less hypercalcemic.

Table **2:** Observational studies examining outcomes associated with VDR agonist therapy in CKD patients

Study	Patients	Therapy	Results
Teng *et al.* [69]	67,399 prevalent hemodialysis patients in the U.S.	Injectable paricalcitol *vs.* calcitriol	16% lower all-cause mortality in the paricalcitol group; improved survival among patients switching from calcitriol to paricalcitol
Shoji *et al.* [71]	242 prevalent hemodialysis patients in Japan	Daily dose of alfacalcidol *vs.* non-users	Reduced mortality from cardiovascular disease in the users; no difference in mortality from non-cardiovascular disease between the two groups
Teng *et al.* [72]	51,037 prevalent hemodialysis patients in the U.S.	Any injectable VDRA *vs.* no treatment	20% lower all-cause mortality in the VDRA group
Melamed *et al.* [73]	1,007 incident hemodialysis and peritoneal dialysis patients in the U.S.	Injectable calcitriol *vs.* no treatment	26% lower all-cause mortality in the calcitriol group *vs.* no treatment
Kalantar-Zadeh *et al.* [74]; Lee *et al.* [75]	58,058 prevalent hemodialysis patients in the U.S.	Injectable paricalcitol *vs.* no treatment	Improved survival associated with any dose of paricalcitol use in time-dependent models
Tentori *et al.* [76]	7731 prevalent hemodialysis patients in the U.S.	Injectable paricalcitol, doxercalciferol or calcitriol *vs.* no treatment	In all models mortality was higher for patients with no VDRA treatment; mortality was similar for paricalcitol *vs.* doxercalciferol; in adjusted models, mortality was not statistically different among 3 VDRAs

Table 2: cont….

Wolf *et al.* [77]	825 incident US hemodialysis patients	Any injectable VDRA *vs.* no treatment	Low vitamin D levels associated with increased mortality; untreated vitamin D deficient patients at significantly increased risk for early mortality
Wolf *et al.* [78]	9303 incident US hemodialysis patients (5110 non-Hispanic white, 979 Hispanic white, 3214 black)	Any injectable VDRA *vs.* no treatment	Treated black patients had 16% lower mortality *vs.* white patients; untreated black patients had 35% higher mortality *vs.* white.
Shinaberger *et al.* [79]	34,307 maintenance hemodialysis patients in the U.S.	Injectable paricalcitol	Higher weekly paricalcitol dosage (normalized by per unit of serum PTH) associated with greater survival
Naves-Diaz *et al.* [80]	Hemodialysis patients (7703 treated *vs.* 8801 untreated) from six Latin America countries	Oral VDRA *vs.* no treatment	Survival advantage observed in the group that had received oral VDRA in 36 of the 37 strata studied including that with the highest levels of serum calcium, phosphorus and PTH
Shoben *et al.* [81]	1,418 nondialysis stages 3 to 4 CKD patients with secondary hyperparathyroidism	Oral calcitriol *vs.* non-users	Oral calcitriol therapy associated with a 26% lower mortality risk and a 20% lower risk for death or dialysis *vs.* non-users.
Kovesdy *et al.* [82]	520 male US veterans with stages 3-5 CKD not on dialysis	Oral calcitriol *vs.* no treatment	Incidence rate ratios for mortality and combined death and dialysis initiation significantly lower in treated patients
Levin *et al.* [83]	4,231 stage 4 CKD patients	Oral VDRA *vs.* no treatment	VDRA use associated with improved survival *vs.* no treatment

VDRA, vitamin D receptor agonist.

However, these studies are rather limited and don't fully explain why different vitamin D analogs behave differently. On the other hand, if indeed different VDRAs do provide differential benefits, especially survival benefits, to CKD patients, then it will be of tremendous interest and importance to find out the mechanism behind the differential effects. Such an understanding will guide the development of new VDRAs with enhanced survival benefits for CKD since currently CKD patients continue to suffer from significantly higher mortality risk than the general public.

Before the mechanism of action for the differential benefits of VDRAs becomes known, the discussion remains at the hypothesis-generating level. However, some observations seem to suggest that the differential effects may have something to do with the differences in therapeutic index for these drugs. It is known from both preclinical and clinical studies that paricalcitol has a 3-4 fold wider therapeutic index than calcitriol. Because of this difference in therapeutic index, paricalcitol can be dosed up to ~10-fold higher than calcitriol. Is it possible that the higher doses of paricalcitol are responsible for its differential benefit in CKD patients?

Wolf *et al.* [78] reported that, in a prospective cohort of non-Hispanic white, Hispanic white, and black incident hemodialysis patients, black patients had 16% lower mortality compared with white patients, but the difference was lost when adjusted for the dosage of VDRAs. In contrast, black patients not treated with any VDRA had 35% higher mortality compared with untreated white patients. They offered an explanation that the survival advantage for Black in dialysis might be due to their receiving more VDRAs because PTH was usually higher among black patients, and consequently they were most likely to receive a higher dose of VDRA.

The recent data from the VITAL clinical trial [57] was particularly interesting. The VITAL study was a double-blind, placebo controlled, multicenter study designed to investigate whether paricalcitol was able to slow CKD progression by measuring on-treatment UACR (Urine Albumin-to-Creatinine Ratio). The last on-treatment UACR for the combined doses of paricalcitol (1 and 2 µg) was lower than that in placebo, but didn't reach a statistical significance. However, the interesting part of the study was that there was a dose-dependent effect of paricalcitol on reducing UACR.

Thus, these observations seem to suggest that the advantage of paricalcitol is associated with its slightly wider therapeutic index than other VDRAs, which allows paricalcitol to be dosed higher, leading to better pleiotropic effects of VDR activation beyond regulation of PTH and mineral homeostasis.

IS THERE A NEED TO DEVELOP NEW FORMS OF VITAMIN D ANALOGS?

VDRA therapy in essence is a hormone replacement therapy that bypasses any potential defect in the complex vitamin D system to activate VDR directly. As discussed in previous chapters, VDR is present in more than 30 tissues and is involved in regulating many functions including the bone, cardiovascular, immune, and renal systems [84, 85]. The endogenous VDR agonist, calcitriol, and its analogs are mainly used to treat SHPT in CKD [44] with some used to treat osteoporosis [86], psoriasis [87] and other diseases. Numerous studies have demonstrated that VDRAs can be used to treat a variety of disorders including kidney and cardiovascular diseases. Yet no VDRAs are indicated for treating kidney or cardiovascular disease, while CKD patients continue to suffer from a high risk of cardiovascular mortality. One key factor limiting the usage of current on-market VDRAs is that current drugs have a narrow (<4-fold) therapeutic index (comparing efficacy *vs.* toxicity) and require frequent dose-titration (changing the drug dosage for the patient based on side effects and efficacy) and serum calcium monitoring (checking the calcium level in the blood). Clinical management using these VDRAs is quite challenging.

If it is true that the pleiotropic effects of VDRAs beyond regulation of PTH and mineral homeostasis depend on their dosages, then VDRAs with a significantly wider therapeutic index than current VDRAs including paricalcitol shall in theory allow for a wider dosing range and greater differential benefits.

What shall be the characteristics of these new VDRAs?

An ideal target product profile for a desirable new VDRM shall include these following characteristics: (1) it should have little or no hypercalcemic toxicity in the efficacious dose range as indicated by biomarkers such as PTH suppression (*i.e.,* a therapeutic window at >10-fold), (2) it should retain the characteristics of the current VDRM chemotype, and (3) it should provide renal and/or cardiovascular protective benefits. The reason for the first criterion is to get away from the need for constant dose titration and serum calcium monitoring. The rationale behind the second criterion is based on the knowledge that a very attractive aspect of the current VDRM chemotype is the apparent lack of other toxicities beside hypercalcemia and the low clinical failure rate for these types of molecules. Since VDR is present in almost every tissue in the human body and is involved in modulating numerous biological and physiological functions, compounds that depart significantly from the current VDRM chemotype may run the risk of evoking off-target toxicities that cannot be easily defined in pre-clinical and/or clinical studies. The reason for the third criterion is supported by current literature and existing data that VDRMs without hypercalcemic toxicity shall bring substantial renal and/or cardiovascular protective benefits to CKD patients receiving the standard of care.

DISCUSSION/CONCLUSION

Review of existing information leads to the conclusion that vitamin D deficiency is linked to various diseases and proper VDR activation is necessary for maintaining good health.

However, even though the vitamin D field has advanced by leaps and bounds during the past decade, many questions remain unanswered. Can it be that a deficiency in VDR activation, not vitamin D and/or 25(OH)D deficiency, is the culprit for various disorders experienced by the general population? In other words, is it possible that there may be a pathological condition called "deficiency in VDR activation" that needs to be treated? If indeed there is such a disease, how shall it be treated? If it can be treated with either vitamin D supplementations or VDRAs, how will one know whether the deficiency in VDR activation has been corrected after therapy? In CKD patients with SHPT, PTH is a useful marker for VDRA therapy. However, if the PTH level is normal, how to gauge whether VDR has been adequately activated after therapy? How about other factors that impact the VDR signaling pathway? Studies have shown that the cutaneous synthesis of vitamin D_3 declines when one ages. Is it possible that the activity of VDR and/or CYP27B1 also goes down during aging? Can it be possible that aging as one of the risk factors for poor health is partially due to deficiency in VDR activation? These questions await answers.

Vitamin D and its analogs are potentially useful for preventing and treating various diseases. However, their usage at this point is still rather limited. It is partially due to the lack of suitable biomarkers to assess the efficacy of vitamin D and its analogs for diseases outside of PTH suppression. Another possible reason is that vitamin D analogs used to treat diseases have narrow therapeutic index and considerable side effects. It will be of tremendous value if biomarkers can be identified and assays developed to determine deficiency in VDR activation. Moreover, new vitamin D analogs that have a wider therapeutic index without the hypercalcemic liability will likely lead to expanded usage of this class of drugs into new applications.

As the field continues to evolve and we develop better understandings of the role of VDR in various biological and pathophysiological functions in the human body, perhaps very soon we will be able to properly diagnose this "deficiency in VDR activation" disease and even develop new ways to treat it.

DISCLOSURE

Part of information in this chapter has been previously published: Wu-Wong, British Journal of Pharmacology Volume 158, Issue 2, pages 395–412, September 2009.

REFERENCES

[1]   Dishmon DA, Dotson JL, Munir A, *et al.* Hypovitaminosis D and valvular calcification in patients with dilated cardiomyopathy. Am J Med Sci 2009; 337:312-316.

[2]   Cuppari L, Garcia-Lopes MG. Hypovitaminosis D in chronic kidney disease patients: prevalence and treatment. J Ren Nutr 2009; 19:38-43.

[3]   Wehr E, Pilz S, Schweighofer N, *et al.* Association of hypovitaminosis D with metabolic disturbances in polycystic ovary syndrome. Eur J Endocrinol 2009; 161:575-582.

[4]   Pilz S, Dobnig H, Winklhofer-Roob B, *et al.* Low serum levels of 25-hydroxyvitamin D predict fatal cancer in patients referred to coronary angiography. Cancer Epidemiol Biomarkers Prev 2008; 17:1228-1233.

[5]   Pierrot-Deseilligny C, Souberbielle JC. Is hypovitaminosis D one of the environmental risk factors for multiple sclerosis? Brain 2010; 133:1869-1888.

[6]   Wu-Wong JR. Potential for vitamin D receptor agonists in the treatment of cardiovascular disease. Br J Pharmacol 2009; 158:395-412.

[7]   Hewison M, Burke F, Evans KN, *et al.* Extra-renal 25-hydroxyvitamin D3-1alpha-hydroxylase in human health and disease. J Steroid Biochem Mol Biol 2007; 103:316-321.

[8]   Andress DL. Vitamin D in chronic kidney disease: a systemic role for selective vitamin D receptor activation. Kidney Int 2006; 69:33-43.

[9]   Jones G. Pharmacokinetics of vitamin D toxicity. Am J Clin Nutr 2008; 88:582S-586S.

[10]   Cranney A, Horsley T, O'Donnell S, *et al.* Effectiveness and safety of vitamin D in relation to bone health. Evid Rep Technol Assess (Full Rep) 2007:1-235.

[11]   Dietary Reference Intakes: Calcium, Phosphorus, Magnesium, Vitamin D, And Fluoride: Washington, DC: National Academy Press, 1997.

[12]   Jackson C, Gaugris S, Sen SS, Hosking D. The effect of cholecalciferol (vitamin D3) on the risk of fall and fracture: a meta-analysis. Qjm 2007; 100:185-192.

[13]   Cannell JJ, Vieth R, Umhau JC, *et al.* Epidemic influenza and vitamin D. Epidemiol Infect 2006; 134:1129-1140.

[14]   Walker VP, Modlin RL. The vitamin D connection to pediatric infections and immune function. Pediatr Res 2009; 65:106R-113R.

[15]   Liu PT, Stenger S, Li H, *et al.* Toll-like receptor triggering of a vitamin D-mediated human antimicrobial response. Science 2006; 311:1770-1773.

[16]   Goldstein MR. Myopathy, statins, and vitamin D deficiency. Am J Cardiol 2007; 100:1328.

[17]   Ceglia L. Vitamin D and its role in skeletal muscle. Curr Opin Clin Nutr Metab Care 2009; 12:628-633.

[18]   Lappe JM, Travers-Gustafson D, Davies KM, Recker RR, Heaney RP. Vitamin D and calcium supplementation reduces cancer risk: results of a randomized trial. Am J Clin Nutr 2007; 85:1586-1591.

[19]   Garland CF, Gorham ED, Mohr SB, Garland FC. Vitamin D for cancer prevention: global perspective. Ann Epidemiol 2009; 19:468-483.

[20]   Peechakara SV, Pittas AG. Vitamin D as a potential modifier of diabetes risk. Nat Clin Pract Endocrinol Metab 2008; 4:182-183.

[21]   Pittas AG, Lau J, Hu FB, Dawson-Hughes B. The role of vitamin D and calcium in type 2 diabetes. A systematic review and meta-analysis. J Clin Endocrinol Metab 2007; 92:2017-2029.

[22]   Lind L, Hanni A, Lithell H, Hvarfner A, Sorensen OH, Ljunghall S. Vitamin D is related to blood pressure and other cardiovascular risk factors in middle-aged men. Am J Hypertens 1995; 8:894-901.

[23]   Canning MO, Grotenhuis K, de Wit H, Ruwhof C, Drexhage HA. 1-alpha,25-Dihydroxyvitamin D3 (1,25(OH)(2)D(3)) hampers the maturation of fully active immature dendritic cells from monocytes. Eur J Endocrinol 2001; 145:351-357.

[24]   Mathieu C, Adorini L. The coming of age of 1,25-dihydroxyvitamin D(3) analogs as immunomodulatory agents. Trends Mol Med 2002; 8:174-179.

[25]   Palomer X, Gonzalez-Clemente JM, Blanco-Vaca F, Mauricio D. Role of vitamin D in the pathogenesis of type 2 diabetes mellitus. Diabetes Obes Metab 2008; 10:185-197.

[26]   Scragg R, Khaw KT, Murphy S. Effect of winter oral vitamin D3 supplementation on cardiovascular risk factors in elderly adults. Eur J Clin Nutr 1995; 49:640-646.

[27]   Pfeifer M, Begerow B, Minne HW, Nachtigall D, Hansen C. Effects of a short-term vitamin D(3) and calcium supplementation on blood pressure and parathyroid hormone levels in elderly women. J Clin Endocrinol Metab 2001; 86:1633-1637.

[28]   Scharla S. [Relative value of plain vitamin D and of biologically active vitamin D in the prevention and treatment of osteoporosis]. Z Rheumatol 2006; 65:391-394, 396-399.

[29]   Richy F, Dukas L, Schacht E. Differential effects of D-hormone analogs and native vitamin D on the risk of falls: a comparative meta-analysis. Calcif Tissue Int 2008; 82:102-107.

[30]   MacLean C, Newberry S, Maglione M, et al. Systematic review: comparative effectiveness of treatments to prevent fractures in men and women with low bone density or osteoporosis. Ann Intern Med 2008; 148:197-213.

[31]   Heist RS, Zhou W, Wang Z, et al. Circulating 25-hydroxyvitamin D, VDR polymorphisms, and survival in advanced non-small-cell lung cancer. J Clin Oncol 2008; 26:5596-5602.

[32]   Li H, Stampfer MJ, Hollis JB, et al. A prospective study of plasma vitamin D metabolites, vitamin D receptor polymorphisms, and prostate cancer. PLoS Med 2007; 4:e103.

[33]   Yang J, Xiong F. [Relevance of CYP27B1 gene promoter polymorphism to autoimmune thyroid diseases]. Nan Fang Yi Ke Da Xue Xue Bao 2008; 28:606-608.

[34]   Lopez ER, Zwermann O, Segni M, et al. A promoter polymorphism of the CYP27B1 gene is associated with Addison's disease, Hashimoto's thyroiditis, Graves' disease and type 1 diabetes mellitus in Germans. Eur J Endocrinol 2004; 151:193-197.

[35]   Holick MF. Vitamin D: importance in the prevention of cancers, type 1 diabetes, heart disease, and osteoporosis. Am J Clin Nutr 2004; 79:362-371.

[36]   Tuohimaa P. Vitamin D and aging. J Steroid Biochem Mol Biol 2009; 114:78-84.

[37]   Lee DM, Rutter MK, O'Neill TW, et al. Vitamin D, parathyroid hormone and the metabolic syndrome in middle-aged and older European men. Eur J Endocrinol 2009; 161:947-954.

[38]   Wortsman J, Matsuoka LY, Chen TC, Lu Z, Holick MF. Decreased bioavailability of vitamin D in obesity. Am J Clin Nutr 2000; 72:690-693.

[39]   Hu XD, Jiang SL, Liu CH, et al. Preventive effects of 1,25-(OH)2VD3 against ConA-induced mouse hepatitis through promoting vitamin D receptor gene expression. Acta Pharmacol Sin 2010; 31:703-708.

[40]   Arteh J, Narra S, Nair S. Prevalence of vitamin D deficiency in chronic liver disease. Dig Dis Sci; 55:2624-2628.

[41]   Petta S, Camma C, Scazzone C, et al. Low vitamin D serum level is related to severe fibrosis and low responsiveness to interferon-based therapy in genotype 1 chronic hepatitis C. Hepatology; 51:1158-1167.

[42]   Targher G, Bertolini L, Scala L, et al. Associations between serum 25-hydroxyvitamin D3 concentrations and liver histology in patients with non-alcoholic fatty liver disease. Nutr Metab Cardiovasc Dis 2007; 17:517-524.

[43]   Levin A, Bakris GL, Molitch M, et al. Prevalence of abnormal serum vitamin D, PTH, calcium, and phosphorus in patients with chronic kidney disease: results of the study to evaluate early kidney disease. Kidney Int 2007; 71:31-38.

[44]   Brown AJ, Slatopolsky E. Drug insight: vitamin D analogs in the treatment of secondary hyperparathyroidism in patients with chronic kidney disease. Nat Clin Pract Endocrinol Metab 2007; 3:134-144.

[45]   Al-Badr W, Martin KJ. Vitamin D and kidney disease. Clin J Am Soc Nephrol 2008; 3:1555-1560.

[46]   Dusso A, Lopez-Hilker S, Rapp N, Slatopolsky E. Extra-renal production of calcitriol in chronic renal failure. Kidney Int 1988; 34:368-375.

[47]   Al-Aly Z, Qazi RA, Gonzalez EA, Zeringue A, Martin KJ. Changes in serum 25-hydroxyvitamin D and plasma intact PTH levels following treatment with ergocalciferol in patients with CKD. Am J Kidney Dis 2007; 50:59-68.

[48]   Zisman AL, Hristova M, Ho LT, Sprague SM. Impact of ergocalciferol treatment of vitamin D deficiency on serum parathyroid hormone concentrations in chronic kidney disease. Am J Nephrol 2007; 27:36-43.

[49]   Panichi V, Migliori M, Taccola D, *et al.* Effects of 1,25(OH)2D3 in experimental mesangial proliferative nephritis in rats. Kidney Int 2001; 60:87-95.

[50]   Tan X, Wen X, Liu Y. Paricalcitol inhibits renal inflammation by promoting vitamin D receptor-mediated sequestration of NF-kappaB signaling. J Am Soc Nephrol 2008; 19:1741-1752.

[51]   Hirata M, Makibayashi K, Katsumata K, *et al.* 22-Oxacalcitriol prevents progressive glomerulosclerosis without adversely affecting calcium and phosphorus metabolism in subtotally nephrectomized rats. Nephrol Dial Transplant 2002; 17:2132-2137.

[52]   Mizobuchi M, Morrissey J, Finch JL, *et al.* Combination therapy with an angiotensin-converting enzyme inhibitor and a vitamin D analog suppresses the progression of renal insufficiency in uremic rats. J Am Soc Nephrol 2007; 18:1796-1806.

[53]   Freundlich M, Quiroz Y, Zhang Z, *et al.* Suppression of renin-angiotensin gene expression in the kidney by paricalcitol. Kidney Int 2008; 74:1394-1402.

[54]   Agarwal R, Acharya M, Tian J, *et al.* Antiproteinuric effect of oral paricalcitol in chronic kidney disease. Kidney Int 2005; 68:2823-2828.

[55]   Alborzi P, Patel NA, Peterson C, *et al.* Paricalcitol reduces albuminuria and inflammation in chronic kidney disease: a randomized double-blind pilot trial. Hypertension 2008; 52:249-255.

[56]   Szeto CC, Chow KM, Kwan BC, Chung KY, Leung CB, Li PK. Oral calcitriol for the treatment of persistent proteinuria in immunoglobulin A nephropathy: an uncontrolled trial. Am J Kidney Dis 2008; 51:724-731.

[57]   de Zeeuw D, Rajiv Agarwal, Michael Amdahl, Paul Audhya, Daniel Coyne, Tushar Garimella, Hans-Henrik Parving, Yili Pritchett, Giuseppe Remuzzi ER, Dennis Andress. Selective vitamin D receptor activation with paricalcitol for reduction of albuminuria in patients with type 2 diabetes (VITAL study): a randomised controlled trial. Lancet 2010; 376:1543-1551.

[58]   Glorieux G, Vanholder R. Blunted response to vitamin D in uremia. Kidney Int Suppl 2001; 78:S182-185.

[59]   Armas LA, Hollis BW, Heaney RP. Vitamin D2 is much less effective than vitamin D3 in humans. J Clin Endocrinol Metab 2004; 89:5387-5391.

[60]   Houghton LA, Vieth R. The case against ergocalciferol (vitamin D2) as a vitamin supplement. Am J Clin Nutr 2006; 84:694-697.

[61]   Slatopolsky E, Finch J, Ritter C, Takahashi F. Effects of 19-nor-1,25(OH)2D2, a new analogue of calcitriol, on secondary hyperparathyroidism in uremic rats. Am J Kidney Dis 1998; 32:S40-47.

[62]   Martin KJ, Gonzalez EA. Vitamin D analogues for the management of secondary hyperparathyroidism. Am J Kidney Dis 2001; 38:S34-40.

[63]   Wu-Wong JR, Noonan W, Ma J, *et al.* Role of phosphorus and vitamin D analogs in the pathogenesis of vascular calcification. J Pharmacol Exp Ther 2006; 318:90-98.

[64]   Henley C, Colloton M, Cattley RC, *et al.* 1,25-Dihydroxyvitamin D3 but not cinacalcet HCl (Sensipar/Mimpara) treatment mediates aortic calcification in a rat model of secondary hyperparathyroidism. Nephrol Dial Transplant 2005; 20:1370-1377.

[65]   Noonan W, Koch K, Nakane M, *et al.* Differential effects of vitamin D receptor activators on aortic calcification and pulse wave velocity in uraemic rats. Nephrol Dial Transplant 2008; 23:3824-3830.

[66]   Cardus A, Panizo S, Parisi E, Fernandez E, Valdivielso JM. Differential effects of vitamin D analogs on vascular calcification. J Bone Miner Res 2007; 22:860-866.

[67]   Mizobuchi M, Finch JL, Martin DR, Slatopolsky E. Differential effects of vitamin D receptor activators on vascular calcification in uremic rats. Kidney Int 2007; 72:709-715.

[68]   Lopez I, Mendoza FJ, Aguilera-Tejero E, *et al.* The effect of calcitriol, paricalcitol, and a calcimimetic on extraosseous calcifications in uremic rats. Kidney Int 2008; 73:300-307.

[69]   Teng M, Wolf M, Lowrie E, Ofsthun N, Lazarus JM, Thadhani R. Survival of patients undergoing hemodialysis with paricalcitol or calcitriol therapy. N Engl J Med 2003; 349:446-456.

[70]   Shoji T, Shinohara K, Kimoto E, *et al.* Lower risk for cardiovascular mortality in oral 1alpha-hydroxy vitamin D3 users in a haemodialysis population. Nephrol Dial Transplant 2004; 19:179-184.

[71]   Teng M, Wolf M, Ofsthun MN, *et al.* Activated injectable vitamin D and hemodialysis survival: a historical cohort study. J Am Soc Nephrol 2005; 16:1115-1125.

[72]   Melamed ML, Eustace JA, Plantinga L, *et al.* Changes in serum calcium, phosphate, and PTH and the risk of death in incident dialysis patients: a longitudinal study. Kidney Int 2006; 70:351-357.

[73]   Kalantar-Zadeh K, Kuwae N, Regidor DL, *et al.* Survival predictability of time-varying indicators of bone disease in maintenance hemodialysis patients. Kidney Int 2006; 70:771-780.

[74]   Lee GH, Benner D, Regidor DL, Kalantar-Zadeh K. Impact of kidney bone disease and its management on survival of patients on dialysis. J Ren Nutr 2007; 17:38-44.

[75]   Tentori F, Hunt WC, Stidley CA, *et al.* Mortality risk among hemodialysis patients receiving different vitamin D analogs. Kidney Int 2006; 70:1858-1865.

[76]   Wolf M, Shah A, Gutierrez O, *et al.* Vitamin D levels and early mortality among incident hemodialysis patients. Kidney Int 2007; 72:1004-1013.

[77]   Wolf M, Betancourt J, Chang Y, *et al.* Impact of activated vitamin D and race on survival among hemodialysis patients. J Am Soc Nephrol 2008; 19:1379-1388.

[78]   Shinaberger CS, Kopple JD, Kovesdy CP, *et al.* Ratio of paricalcitol dosage to serum parathyroid hormone level and survival in maintenance hemodialysis patients. Clin J Am Soc Nephrol 2008; 3:1769-1776.

[79]   Naves-Diaz M, Alvarez-Hernandez D, Passlick-Deetjen J, *et al.* Oral active vitamin D is associated with improved survival in hemodialysis patients. Kidney Int 2008; 74:1070-1078.

[80]   Shoben AB, Rudser KD, de Boer IH, Young B, Kestenbaum B. Association of oral calcitriol with improved survival in nondialyzed CKD. J Am Soc Nephrol 2008; 19:1613-1619.

[81]   Kovesdy CP, Ahmadzadeh S, Anderson JE, Kalantar-Zadeh K. Association of activated vitamin D treatment and mortality in chronic kidney disease. Arch Intern Med 2008; 168:397-403.

[82]   Levin A, Djurdjev O, Beaulieu M, Er L. Variability and risk factors for kidney disease progression and death following attainment of stage 4 CKD in a referred cohort. Am J Kidney Dis 2008; 52:661-671.

[83]   Nakane M, Ma J, Rose AE, Osinski MA, Wu-Wong JR. Differential effects of Vitamin D analogs on calcium transport. J Steroid Biochem Mol Biol 2007; 103:84-89.

[84]   de Borst MH, de Boer R, Stolk RP, Slaets JP, Wolffenbuttel BH, Navis G. Vitamin D Deficiency: Universal Risk Factor for Multifactorial Diseases? Curr Drug Targets 2011; 12(1):97-106.

[85]   Holick MF. The vitamin D deficiency pandemic and consequences for nonskeletal health: mechanisms of action. Mol Aspects Med 2008; 29:361-368.

[86]   Cheskis BJ, Freedman LP, Nagpal S. Vitamin D receptor ligands for osteoporosis. Curr Opin Investig Drugs 2006; 7:906-911.

[87]   Fogh K, Kragballe K. New vitamin D analogs in psoriasis. Curr Drug Targets Inflamm Allergy 2004; 3:199-204.

Index

www.ingramcontent.com/pod-product-compliance
Lightning Source LLC
Chambersburg PA
CBHW041717210326

41598CB00007B/688